LOOK GREAT
NATURALLY

...Without Ditching the Lipstick

JANEY LEE GRACE

HAY HOUSE

Australia • Canada • Hong Kong • India
South Africa • United Kingdom • United States

Fi~~rst published and~~ ~~United Kingdom by:~~
~~Hay House UK Ltd~~ ~~W10 5BE~~
Tel.: (4~~4) 20 8962 1230; Fax: (44) 20 8962 1239. www.hayhouse.~~~~c~~~~~~uk

Pu~~blished and distributed in the United States of America by:~~
Hay House, Inc., ~~PO Box 5100~~ ~~A 92018-51~~~~(1) 760 43~~ ~~695 or (800)~~
654 512 ~~(1) 760 431 6948; (800) 650 5115. www.hayhouse.c~~~~om~~

~~Published and distributed in Australia by:~~
Hay House Aust~~ralia Ltd, 18/36 Ralph St, Alexandria NSW 2015. Tel.: (61) 2~~ 9669 4299;
Fax: (61) 2 9669 4144. www.hayhouse.com.au

Published and distributed in the Republic of South Africa by:
Hay House SA (Pty), Ltd, PO Box 990, Witkoppen 2068.
Tel./Fax: (27) 11 467 8904. www.hayhouse.co.za

Published and distributed in India by:
Hay House Publishers India, Muskaan Complex, Plot No.3, B–2, Vasant Kunj, New Delhi –
110 070. Tel.: (91) 11 4176 1620; Fax: (91) 11 4176 1630. www.hayhouse.co.in

Distributed in Canada by:
Raincoast, 9050 Shaughnessy St, Vancouver, BC V6P 6E5.
Tel.: (1) 604 323 7100; Fax: (1) 604 323 2600

© Janey Lee Grace, 2010

The moral rights of the author have been asserted.

The author of this book does not dispense medical advice or prescribe the use of any technique
as a form of treatment for physical or medical problems without the advice of a physician,
either directly or indirectly. The intent of the author is only to offer information of a general
nature to help you in your quest for emotional and spiritual well-being. In the event you use
any of the information in this book for yourself, which is your constitutional right, the author
and the publisher assume no responsibility for your actions.

A catalogue record for this book is available from the British Library.

ISBN 978-1-84850-203-1

Printed and bound in Great Britain by
TJ International, Padstow, Cornwall.

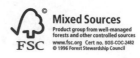

Mixed Sources
Product group from well-managed
forests and other controlled sources
www.fsc.org Cert no. SGS-COC-2482
© 1996 Forest Stewardship Council

Contents

Acknowledgements

Motivational... inspirational... creative... knowledge-able.... encouraging... loving... those who contributed to this book, some of them own personal mentors and very dear friends Enid, Glenn, Glenn, Aly, Dawn, Ken, Jason, Tabitha, Tej, Petre, Mariano, Abigail, Matt, and all my wonderful forum members at www.imperfectlynatural.com – and not forgetting all the incredible natural companies who are recommended here.

Supportive... enthusiastic... understanding... on the case... always nagging (nicely!)... my agent Tony and all at Hay House, especially Jo, Jo, Joanna, Michelle and Carolyn, thanks also to freelance editor Barbara.

Joyful... cheeky... exuberant... driving me bananas... exhausting... gorgeous... my four beautiful children who got mighty fed up with 'mummy always on the 'puter'.

My rock... the wind beneath and all that... I couldn't have done any of it without my divine hubby Simon.

Introduction

Do you want to look and feel fantastic? Not just once or twice a year when you're off on your summer holiday or treating yourself to a facial before a big bash, but just about all of the time? How would it be if your skin glowed, your hair shone, you were at your optimum weight and you had incredible energy and vitality? Your friends asking constantly, 'What are you on?' and wanting to get some, too? How about if your new lifestyle was really simple to achieve, saved you copious amounts of money, released you from needing to trawl the cosmetic counters in department stores and, as if that weren't enough, let you feel just a teeny bit smug because you'd be a couple of shades greener, not through any major eco-effort but simply by embracing a healthy, natural and organic lifestyle?

This book is all over it. It's about how to look and feel great while still being glam, saving money *and* doing our bit for the planet. Enlightened gals, by doffing their berets (green, of course) to holistic living, are making sustainable choices *and* doing their bit for the planet – almost without trying.

Many girls recycle their shopping bags, buy Ecover washing-up liquid and try a bit of 'carbon off-setting' but are still burdening their skin with scary chemicals, sleeping badly, and consuming those hidden e-numbers. Your clothes may be Fairtrade, but what chemicals are they treated with? And, most importantly, do you look good in them? I hope to prove that the words 'beauty', 'fashion', 'style' – and, indeed, 'joy' and 'simplicity' – can be linked with the word 'natural' without making you think of sackcloth!

KEEPING IT SIMPLE

Beauty comes from health, confidence, contentment and making the best of what you've got, and there's a way to get there – organically and naturally. You don't have to be a fashion victim to care about the clothes you wear; you don't have to be a drop-dead gorgeous model to want to make the most of your looks. Our personal style is intrinsic to who we are. Others judge us on what we choose to wear and, with or without make-up, something about an expression on your face can convey more than words.

The ideas in this book offer you, the modern, savvy girl-friend, freedom from the 'consumer trap'. There are inspirational tips for a joyful, more carefree life, and tons of great ideas for ditching the guilt around recycling your rubbish, doing the housework, and coveting the latest disposable fashion item or designer perfume. Alongside this there is advice about which water we should all be drinking and sensible guidance on diets, exercise and how to stay well without going near a pharmacy.

I want to remind you urban, sassy gals that you're already gorgeous, and help you tap into who you are. I've got no intention of ditching my lust for sparkly gold eye shadow and nail polish – but I've discovered (and will share with you), where to get organic mineral make-up and formaldehyde-free varnish. I'll stress that nature has actually provided everything we need and, instead of popping a pill, there are simple kitchen cupboard remedies for when you're feeling full of cold or the kids have chicken pox. I'll look at how to help along that process of 'finding yourself' with the assistance of life-coaching, shamanic healing and positive visualization techniques. I'll cover mind, body and spirit from a very 'accessible' perspective, and ask if it really is possible to use cosmic ordering to get what we desire.

Throughout the book there are also a fantastic bunch of top 'secrets' from a variety of girlfriends who are happy to share their experiences and wisdom with you.

KEEPING IT REAL

Look Great Naturally... Without Ditching the Lipstick is also about living a little more simply, in the style of Oliver James' *Affluenza* and Tom Hodgkinson's *How to Be Idle* and *How to Be Free*. This book looks at this message from a female perspective – in the knowledge that it's time to chill a little and find beauty in the now. It also takes a leaf from Carl Honore's *In Praise of Slow* and looks at the slow movement as it spreads (slowly!) across the UK.

The economic climate has made many of us re-evaluate our priorities. In many cases that means having less money to spend and trying to create more time for things that really matter, like working out what you really want, making time for family and friends, thinking about your contribution to your community and not forgetting assessing the size of your carbon footprint. But rather than get all serious and just lecture you, I'm offering a wealth of ideas – delivered with my sense of humour intact – and a truly fast-track approach to 'having it all' while still embracing the natural alternative. That means you can simplify a little, save money and the planet, while still hanging on to that all-important lipstick!

I am passionate about living holistically but I'm by no means an old-school 'knit your own yoghurt' sandal-wearing Earth Mother. I'm a working mum with four kids under 11 and, somehow, I seem to have found a balance, albeit imperfectly, in the maelstrom of madness that is working in the media, being a wife and mum and running the website imperfectlynatural.com. On that note I am so grateful also to my 24/7 forum of like-minded 'girlfriends', all exchanging tips through the night and eagerly trying my latest recommendations for anything natural, especially if it doesn't (in any sense) cost the earth. Our discussions and forums have been a great inspiration for me in writing this book.

IMPERFECTLY NATURAL

I hope these ideas will appeal to you whether you've always been a passionate 'eco-warrior' or if you're new to the field of combat. Even the affluent 'ladies who lunch' can find they enjoy the natural path to health, well-being and happiness. This book is of course my own, very personal account of trying to look and feel great naturally, but I promise I won't be preachy. In some instances I've simply done some of the research and groundwork for you, while in others I'm just offering up the question, happy to admit honestly that I also still have much to learn in my quest for a holistic life. I've always called my trip down this road an *im*perfectly natural one, because I admit to not getting it all right. It's the 'small change/big difference' approach.

ONE SMALL CHANGE

Feel free to dip in and out wherever it appeals to you – and if at any point you feel overwhelmed, just decide to start with one small change. Switch your deodorant to a natural one, perhaps, or pop a protective device on your mobile phone, or try swapping your usual lunch for a superfood salad. Whatever it is, start slowly – holistic living wasn't built in a day!

Talking food, by the way, I aim to encourage you to get 'in the raw'. By that I'm not saying that you must give up your lovely cooked foods forever, but I'm going to persuade you that eating a high percentage of really yummy raw foods and fresh juices will make a tremendous difference to how great you feel – and look.

Now let's get gorgeous … naturally!

Janey's Guide to Skincare

This book will change your skincare regime.

'Oh, please,' I hear you cry – 'don't scare me with tales of how my favourite light-reflective concealer contains evil nano-particles!'

OK, I promise I won't name and shame brands – but I guarantee I'll show you some wicked alternatives to everything from nail polish without formaldehyde to hair dye without resorcinol – if the chemical names don't mean much to you, don't worry, just trust me: you can remain gorgeous, feeling pampered and full of health without ditching the lipstick (or, indeed, any product you usually buy to enhance your considerable natural beauty). You'll also be able to tick the no animal cruelty, Fairtrade and eco boxes without even trying. Result!

Recent market research reports show that the rise in spending on organic skincare products has gone up by at least 40 per cent, so undoubtedly many of us are starting to consider what's in the skincare products we buy.

OUTSIDE IN

Let's not forget that our skin is the largest organ in our body, and that what we put on it goes inside it, too. Scientists reckon that at least 60 per cent of creams, lotions and potions, etc. that are applied topically (on the skin) are ingested into our bodies. Of course, individual ingredients vary as to the extent they can penetrate the layers of the skin. It's thought that the average girlfriend will absorb 5 lb worth of potentially toxic chemicals through personal care products annually. It's not a pleasant thought, but to pick out just one chemical – formaldehyde (yep, the stuff in those jars in science class used to preserve animal remains!) is found in deodorants, nail polishes and even shower gels. Embalmers report that they now can often find 50 per cent more of this chemical in dead bodies than they did 10 years ago.

When I was younger I was convinced that so long as I removed my make-up at the end of the day, I'd come to no harm. Then I realized that both creams and skin patches are used in hormone replacement therapy. It was a wake-up call. If one small amount of cream can disrupt an entire menstrual cycle, then it's clear that the copious amounts of creams, lotions, moisturizers, gels, etc. in our personal care products can absolutely have an impact on our physical and even our emotional health.

It's a good idea to check the ingredients on your skin-care products just as thoroughly as you check for e-numbers, colours and preservatives in foods. But what should you be looking for?

I suggest looking for what's NOT in there rather than what is. A product may well say 'organic' on the label, but that may apply to only one ingredient. I came across a bottle of 'organic' aloe vera shampoo: it contained 2 per cent organic aloe vera, while the remaining 98 per cent was a mix of chemicals that I decided I'd rather *not* put on my scalp! Ethical skincare companies who really are natural will lay out their credentials proudly, usually stating on their packaging that their products contain no SLSs (sodium laurel sulphates), parabens, preservatives, artificial fragrances or phthalates. All of those shouldn't be found anywhere on a so-called 'natural' product, but because they're usually disguised in very long chemical names it can be hard to know. That's why it's easier to look for labels that make it clear they don't include any nasties.

Of course, if a skincare or beauty product is 100 per cent organic, you're onto a winner. I'll recommend a few ranges later in this chapter. Products certified organic by the Soil Association, Ecocert or BDIH are also usually pretty exemplary, as in order to achieve those important accreditations a company will have had to invest a considerable amount of money and effort in their ethical credentials.

Be warned, though, that the words 'natural', 'dermatologically tested', 'hypoallergenic' and even the aforementioned 'organic' are rather meaningless and can be used as a marketing tool to try and persuade you into thinking a product is natural because it contains one organic or natural ingredient. You need to be wary, but after reading this book you should have one up on the powerful marketing guys who think they can fool you into paying a fortune for skincare that claims to rejuvenate your skin or remove wrinkles while the chemicals it contains can do you more harm than good.

Dr Mariano Spiezia is a homeopathic doctor and founder of the UK's first range of 100 per cent organic skincare. He has this to say about our skin:

The skin is a true organ of the body, intimately linked to and an integral part of the whole, and whose state of health or disease it so eloquently reveals, like a mirror reflecting the body's innermost workings. Among its many functions it acts both as an emunctory – detox – organ, expelling toxins from the body, as well as a respiratory organ capable of absorbing oxygen and releasing CO_2. A real external lung!

Therefore the beauty of the skin is also an expression of its health, which is largely dependent on the health of the body within. We owe it to ourselves and to our skin to keep it well nourished, cleansed and detoxed from both inside and out.

If your skincare is labelled organic, check for accreditation.

– The Soil Association is the main UK accrediting body. For a product to be labelled 'organic', at least 95 per cent of the ingredients must be organic: www.soilassociation.org

– Alternatively, if 70 per cent of the ingredients are organic, the labelling must state the ingredients and percentages.

- The Organic Farmers and Growers Association is another source of information: www.organicfarmers.org.uk

- Many of the products sold in the UK are accredited by the German accreditation body BDIH: www.bdih.de

- The French accrediting body Ecocert: www.ecocert.com

CHEMICAL WARFARE

'So what's wrong with my regular designer brand of skincare?' I hear you cry. 'I've used it for years, and it's the only one that doesn't bring me out in hives ...' Well, that may be so, but let me remind you that most conventional products are petroleum-based – in other words, effectively hazardous waste! Of course that wouldn't smell, look or feel very nice, so added to that heady mix is usually:

- sodium laurel sulphate, a detergent known to cause irritation
- artificial fragrances known to cause headaches, fatigue and insomnia
- parabens, preservatives which, when they combine, can cause all manner of problems.

It gets tricky when you realize that even some so-called 'natural' and 'organic' brands use high-foaming detergents in their shampoos and body washes. Many allegedly perfectly 'safe' and licensed-for-use synthetic chemicals can have hormone-disrupting potential. Certain preservatives mimic the hormone oestrogen in the body, and could therefore be linked to breast cancer.

Every day, it's estimated we put more than 500 different chemicals on our bodies, all in the name of beauty. Even a dab of perfume can contain 200 different substances in one go! Often these are artificial fragrances that are irritating to the skin, and repeated exposure means a person can become 'sensitized' and develop an allergic reaction.

The environmental group Safe Cosmetics says:

> *More than one-third of all personal care products*
> *contain at least one ingredient linked to cancer. When*
> *risky and unstudied chemicals are used in cosmetics,*
> *the stakes can be high ... Research shows there may be*
> *long-term, gradual effects linked to chemical ingredients*
> *used in cosmetics. The components of a product are not*
> *trace contaminants like those found at parts-per-million*
> *or even parts-per-billion levels in food and water. These*
> *are the base ingredients of the product, just as flour is an*
> *ingredient in bread. We are finding that many chemicals*
> *associated with health hazards are stored and accumu-*
> *late in the body, many passing onto unborn children.*
>
> *– www.safecosmetics.org*

Of course, no single jar of moisturizer, tube of mascara or bottle of shampoo or indeed perfume is going to cause fatigue or insomnia, exacerbate eczema, allergies or contribute to Alzheimer's disease or cancer, but the cumulative effect of the thousands of different chemicals packed into our many different products almost certainly will. Over time, toxic chemicals can build up in our tissues and be stored in our body fat or our liver, although of course it would be hard to prove they are to blame for our chronic or even acute conditions.

Individually, of course, all chemicals used in beauty, skincare and cleaning products are legal and passed as safe. It's usually deemed that a small amount of toxins is acceptable because they are at such a low dose. Some people may even argue that chemicals are tested so rigorously that indeed they're safer than many natural ingredients. The issue is, however, what happens when sheer force of numbers come into the equation. Our mums and grandmas most probably owned one pot of cold cream and a nice rich red lipstick, perhaps a hair spray, but that would have been about it. They certainly would not have had 30 different make-up items, another 30 or 50 different products in the bathroom, and yet another 25 under the kitchen sink. In the name of progress we've complicated everything so that we're almost swimming in a kind of chemical soup – and a huge number of different products equates to a huge number of chemicals which, when they interact, can become toxic, even carcinogenic.

It's impossible to do the calculations because there are an estimated 100,000 synthetic chemicals licensed for use now, with a further thousand coming onto the marketplace each year. It's estimated that over 10,000 chemicals are used in our skincare products, so clearly it's not possible to test what happens when chemical license number 453 is placed alongside 236 and 189 and then left in direct sunlight!

THE ALTERNATIVE

Let's get back to the good news. The growth in choice in the organic, ethical and natural market is massive and there's a wealth of affordable choice available. You can also, of course, be even more chic and make your own personalized concoctions. See pages 38–51 for some recipes and suggestions.

Let's start with the recommended ethical, natural skincare companies. Fortunately there are masses now competing for your cash. Here are just a few of my favourites, but I suggest you check my website regularly for the latest offers and new companies. You can also buy most of the products I recommend at www.janeysnaturalstore.com.

Many natural companies are small operations, often just a girlfriend disillusioned by what she's seen on sale, who decides to make her own, gives a few bottles away as gifts to friends and, before long, has a thriving small business. But the bigger, more established companies include:

- www.weleda.co.uk
- www.greenpeople.co.uk
- www.lavera.co.uk
- www.faithinnature.co.uk
- www.drbronner.com
- www.kinetic4health.co.uk

You'll find their products in health shops as well as online. They're excellent, with a large range of affordable, ethical, cruelty-free products.

A few special companies are unique in that their small ranges are 100 per cent organic:

- www.inlight-online.co.uk. Inlight is run, as mentioned earlier, by Dr Mariano Spiezia.

- Dr Spiezia was also the original founder of the UK's first-ever range of 100 per cent organic skincare: www.spieziaorganics.com
- www.balmbalm.co.uk
- www.badgerbalm.com

There are also many smaller operations, whose products are mostly sold online or in small health shops or holistic salons. A huge amount of care and attention have gone into these products and there's often an interesting story around why the company was founded. To mention just a few:

- www.elenasnaturecollection.co.uk
- www.purenuffstuff.co.uk
- www.sensitiveskincareco.com
- www.naturalskincarecompany.com
- www.jowoodorganics.com
- www.essential-care.co.uk
- www.herbfarmacy.co.uk
- www.lucyrose.biz
- www.lucyrussellorganics.com
- www.beyondskincare.co.uk
- www.raw-ganic.com
- www.akamuti.co.uk

For natural soaps and bathtime products:

- www.trevarnoskincare.com
- www.handmadenaturals.co.uk

Girlfriends' Natural Secrets ... Put your cream on with upward strokes; have a positive attitude to life – it will show in your face and eyes; and drink water!

– Jenny Seagrove

IN THE RAW

A few companies now offer 'raw skincare'. Yep, just as with raw foods, the live enzymes remain intact in these beauty products. Raw skincare uses ingredients that are not pasteurized or processed and aren't heated to more than 40°C. This is significant because heating oils is thought to create free radicals, those pesky molecules that mix with oxygen to turn apples brown and age our skin (inside and out). Free radicals damage collagen and result in wrinkles.

Live Native (www.livenative.com) claim that their organic ingredients are either unrefined or unpasteurized, and carefully sourced either for their raw state or the low temperatures used in extracting and processing them. Their creams are blended without heat, which means the naturally occurring goodies (antioxidants, essential fatty acids and active healing plant matter) remain intact.

Raw Gaia (www.rawgaia.com) is another small UK-based company which has developed the first 'living' skincare range using only cold-pressed, organic and vegan ingredients.

Yet again, if you have a bunch of raw ingredients, a mortar and pestle and perhaps a high-speed blender, it's pretty easy to concoct your own raw skincare products. See recipes later (beginning on page 33).

MOISTURIZING

Shea butter, apricot kernel oil, aloe vera and coconut oils are often used in live skincare for their wonderful rehydrating qualities.

Coconut Oil

It's fair to say I'm a huge fan of coconut oil particularly – it has so many benefits, both for nutrition and for skincare. It's been categorized as a 'functional' food because it's absorbed directly by the liver and so its calories are burned off more quickly than calories from other fat sources. (This is why some people use it as an aid to weight loss.) It's extremely high in lauric acid, one of the main ingredients in breast-milk! It's also anti-bacterial and high in calcium, potassium and iron, and helps with the absorption of minerals. It has been used by athletes including the England rugby team, because it assists in raising the body's metabolic rate and therefore helps the body burn fat adequately. It can protect us against bacteria and infections. It's a great oil to use for frying as it doesn't degrade at high temperatures. I keep a tub by the cooker – and another by the bath, as it's also one of the cheapest and best moisturizers you'll find. It heals, moisturizes and protects all skin types.

I'd highly recommend Coconoil virgin coconut oil, which is a Fairtrade product from Sri Lanka (www.coconoil.com). If you haven't used it before you may be surprised to find when you open the tub it looks like white lard, solidifying in cold temperatures. At room temperature it is a liquid. Keep a long-handled teaspoon nearby and as soon as you put a blob of it on the palm of your hand it will turn to oil and you can use it as you would any other body oil. You can also put a spoonful straight into your bathwater which makes it soft and silky and means you need to use less after bathing. Coconut oil is great for adding to the bathwater for children or babies. It's wonderfully nourishing for hands and feet and, so long as a night of passion isn't on the cards(!), last thing at night smother your hands and feet in it, put on cotton gloves/socks, and in the morning you'll feel the difference. One tub lasts for ages.

Coconut oil also makes a fantastic hair-conditioning treatment. Leave it on overnight (same as the hand and foot treatment) if you really want to be soft and silky the next day. Just make sure you give it a couple of washes the next morning. For a quick conditioning hair mask, add a teaspoon of honey to a couple of tablespoons of coconut oil and leave for ten minutes, then wash out.

If you're worried you're going to smell like some coconut-y beach babe, virgin coconut oil actually doesn't have a strong smell at all. Your memory of that heavy coconut smell probably originates from using sun lotions which contain artificial fragrances but have never been near a real coconut! If on the other hand you actually like a bit of fragrance, simply add a few drops of essential oil to a small amount of coconut oil, or try one of the DIY recipes listed later in this chapter. For a really luxurious treat, get yourself a pot of gardenia-scented coconut oil from Sensitive Skincare (www.sensitiveskincareco.com).

Girlfriends' Natural Secrets ... Coconut oil for anywhere on my body, even to clean and moisturize my face. Also after a bath I file the hard skin on my feet, then give them a good massage with coconut oil and put on a clean pair of socks for the night so the oil can soak in.

Girlfriends' Aspirations ... To be able to do cartwheels even though I never learned how to do them as a child.

– Michele Kaye, Nia teacher www.nianow.com

Girlfriends' Natural Secrets ... *I always use organic rosehip oil on my face. It is excellent for the very sensitive skin around the eyes and I am convinced it helps with those little lines that seem to increase with age!*

Girlfriends' Aspirations ... *I would love a natural talent – to play the piano beautifully or to be able to draw. Unfortunately I can't do either!*
  – Soo Cieszynska, sales manager Synergy Products

BATHTIME

While we're on the subject of bathwater, by the way, to soften skin you can dissolve a tablespoon of honey into the bathwater and try the 'oat bag remedy'. Simply get a small muslin bag or thin sock, fill it with porridge oats and tie it at the top. You can wet it and use as a wash mitt or hang it from the tap and run the water through it; the bathwater will turn milky and you'll feel rather like Cleopatra bathing in milk. It will soothe any itchy or irritated skin (can be used for children or adults).

If you're feeling creative you can add some sprigs of lavender or rose petals to the bag or even put a few drops of your favourite essential oil directly on the bag or sock. The bath will smell heavenly.

Avoid regular bubble baths and those conventional bath cubes or 'bombs'. Remember you can get a natural version of everything. For gorgeous shea butter fizzing bath 'bombs' see www.potions.com. You can also make your own bathtime treats and of course any bathtime will become a relaxing experience if you simply add a few drops of essential oil (we'll talk more about essential oils later on).

NATURAL HOME SPA
To create your own home spa experience, simply clear your diary for a few hours, switch off your phone and enjoy some self-indulgent natural pampering.

Set the Mood
Create the right mood, have some fresh bath towels to hand (for organic cotton or bamboo towels, see www.diva-stores.com and www.ethicalsuperstore.com) and if it's evening light some candles. It's worth spending a little while making your bathroom inviting, even if it's only by adding candlelight and a few pretty shells that remind you of your hols!

Skin-brushing
Start by dry skin-brushing. Invest in a good bristle brush and work in small circular movements, upwards from your feet. This should tingle a bit but not be painful. You'll find over time you'll be able to build up to using more pressure. This is incredible for improving circulation and helping to remove toxins. It can also help with cellulite. Girlfriends of mine have reported that the appearance of cellulite is massively decreased after a couple of weeks of daily skin-brushing. Can't be bad! This happens because if you do it right it can help boost collagen production, which helps the elasticity of the skin.

Starting from your feet, work upwards in circular movements. Literally cover every bit of your body, including the soles of your feet and the insides and backs of each leg. Go very gently across your stomach in tiny circular movements, and brush gently downwards under your arms around the important lymph area. A good time to do this is just before a shower, then afterwards dry yourself off and apply body moisturizer as usual.

A Word About Cellulite

If cellulite is a real issue for you, you'll have read about many products claiming to banish cellulite or at least reduce the appearance of the annoying orange-peel skin, including tights that claim to massage away cellulite, tights that contain minerals extracted from marine plants (Thalassotherapy tights) and support tights that work on compression. There are also tights impregnated with caffeine which are said to boost the metabolism. None of the above float my boat, but then I'm not a fan of those control-top tights or pants either – they always feel as though they're cutting off your blood supply! – but they shouldn't do you any harm if you fancy trying them.

What I would recommend, though, is to take the 'caffeine tights' approach but make it simpler and cheaper – use coffee grounds! Put a few spoonfuls of used coffee grounds onto a damp sponge and, using big circular movements, massage your thighs and legs. Let's face it, on whether caffeine really does help to burn fat and diminish the appearance of cellulite the jury's out, but using it this way sure is better for you than drinking it!

Other tips for combating cellulite include drinking lots of citrus juice and applying citrus essential oils such as lemon and lime. Mix with a carrier oil and massage all around the area. Weleda's birch cellulite oil is good, it's a unique combination of plant extracts and natural plant oils which visibly improves the skin's texture and smoothness by stimulating the body's own regulating and regenerating processes. They are able to claim great results after only a month's use (www.weleda.co.uk).

For other natural cellulite treatments check out the Essential Oil Company (www.eoco.org.uk). And try the excellent Ultimate Beauty Skin Repair Oil (100 per cent organic) from www.viridian-nutrition.com.

Skin health

Inside: *Choose a predominantly vegetarian and organic diet, rich in vitamins and minerals. Drink enough water to make your urine clear in colour. In addition to the antioxidant vitamins 'par excellence' – A, E and C – and the essential fatty acids omega 3 and omega 6, your skin also needs sulphur and silica to keep collagen and elastin in good health.*

You will find sulphur in asparagus, onions, garlic, watercress, rocket, Brussels sprouts, pulses, wholegrains and yeast flake. You will find silica in cucumber, asparagus, parsley, millet, rye, Jerusalem artichokes, brown rice, potatoes and horsetail. Twice a year, in spring and autumn as the seasons change, drink daily for a month 2–3 cups of nettle, horsetail, calendula and lemon verbena tea, to which you have added 20 drops of burdock and 15 of heartsease tinctures.

Out: *Whilst you shower, stimulate the skin's circulation by gently scrubbing the body all over with a mitten of natural plant fibre to help the skin oxygenate itself and* *improve its metabolic exchange. After you shower, add a handful of Himalayan salts to a hot bath and soak for 20 minutes. The salts will help the skin to release waste and toxins, leaving your skin squeaky clean. Finish off by massaging your whole body with a 100 per cent organic body oil formulated from the purest plant-based, cold-pressed oils and herbal extracts, to give your skin proper nourishment and all the precious essential fatty acids for its good health.*

Dr Mariano Spiezia, www.inlight-online.com

Hydrotherapy

If you've been lucky enough to go to Champneys or one of the other UK or European spas that offer hydrotherapy, you'll know it's an incredibly stimulating treatment. So once you've done your dry skin-brushing, give yourself a mini-Kneipp session. Hydrotherapy is sometimes called Kneipp after the Bavarian monk who first discovered that water has healing properties. He immersed his body in ice-cold water daily, and cured himself of a serious illness. Now, I don't fancy that much, but it's worth trying to kick-start your circulation by alternating cold and hot water. Get a bowl of each, sit on a stool and put your feet first into the cold water – this makes your blood vessels contract and stimulates everything – then put your feet immediately into the hot water (as hot as you can bear comfortably); this dilates the blood vessels and helps you to begin to shed toxins.

If you've ever tried the freezing cold plunge-pool at the sauna, the theory is the same. At home you can have a quick dip in a bath of cold water before taking a hot shower.

At the very least, it's worth having a quick blast of cold water after a hot shower to close the pores. It's definitely invigorating!

Self-massage

In addition to skin-brushing, it's great to spend some time doing some massage on yourself. This helps to stimulate circulation and relieve aches and pains. Simply use small circular movements or grab a massage tool if you need to reach your middle back. You can use one of those long-handled brushes or even an old style 'back scratcher'.

It's easy to give yourself a relaxing foot massage: make firm, stroking movements along the sole of your foot from ankle to toes, then hold a foot with one hand and make small circular movements with your thumb down the sole, applying firm pressure to the ball of the foot. Stroke individual toes firmly, paying attention to the very end of each toe to stimulate energy flow.

Scented Bath

Once you've given yourself some TLC, relax in a bath scented with essential oils and breathe deeply. Use this time to think only healing thoughts.

Girlfriends' Natural Secrets ... This is courtesy of my still beautiful mother – instead of moisturizer at bedtime, cover your face with live yogurt made from goat's milk – not too much, of course, or your partner will not be best pleased! It has an amazing effect on the skin, making it softer, smoother and much clearer. Persevere, as it takes a couple of weeks for the effect to really kick in. I'm a recent convert but my mother has done this for years, and even in her mid-70s she can still give Joan Collins a run for her money!

Girlfriends' Aspirations ... Repeat this affirmation

– 'I live in an oasis of calm, meditating daily in a beautiful, draped white room, somewhere high in the mountains – the sounds I can hear are the wind and gentle tinkling of bells and wind chimes, not four kids battling and screaming, competing with a permanently ringing phone. My head is full of peace instead of to-do lists, my body is slender, toned and bursting with life and vitality, not weary, aching and constantly craving chocolate ... I am serenity personified.'

– Carolyn Von Outersterp,
www.jollydaysluxurycamping.co.uk

DEODORANTS

If you've never considered natural alternatives before, buying a natural deodorant is a good place to start. What's wrong with the conventional ones? Well ... *everything*.

Many oncologists in breast cancer units now tell their patients to avoid conventional deodorants, largely due to the incidences of unusually high levels of aluminium being found in the breast tissue of women with cancer. Some may argue that it's merely 'trace elements' of aluminium from the food and drink we consume, but even if that were the case, which I doubt, I would argue that women definitely do *not* need artificial fragrances, alcohol, propylene glycol (a crude oil also found in brake fluid) or parabens and pre-servatives – all found in conventional deodorizing products. Recent studies show that in 80 per cent of breast cancer cases, parabens are found in the tissue.

Avoid anti-perspirants at all cost. Our bodies are designed to perspire and clear the toxins, and as the underarm area is very sensitive and linked to the lymphatic system, we need to *encourage* the release of toxins to keep the immune system strong. Blocking the pores could make it more difficult for the body to fight infection.

Interestingly, over the years I've found that the better my diet, the less I need any deodorant at all. When I did my first juice detox retreat, I forgot to take my natural deodorant with me. I'd been eating fairly healthily for a couple of weeks to build up to it, and I found that even though I was doing lots of exercise in high temperatures I didn't feel I needed to ask to borrow a deodorant – I simply didn't smell bad! And honestly, I don't think I was just kidding myself, because I asked several other people whether it had affected them that way and most said they had applied some deodorant almost out of habit but in fact they hadn't been conscious of their sweat being as whiffy as usual. I assume this can only be because the purer your diet, the less pungent the toxins being released. I now find if I drink lots of coffee and alcohol, and go back on the processed and spicy foods, I need deodorant – but if I juice regularly and have a high proportion of fresh raw foods, I don't need any.

Mineral Deodorants

While you're just getting started on this road, though, opt for deodorants that are free from synthetic chemicals, aluminium chlorohydrate and petroleum. Choose one that is 100 per cent natural and vegan. To start with, you could try a natural 'crystal' deodorant. These come in the form of roll-ons in handy packaging and are incredibly good value. Most health shops stock them now. The ingredient listed is usually just potassium alum, and the theory is that you rub it gently onto wet skin and it leaves a fine layer of mineral salts. Don't worry, you can't see or smell them and, fortunately, you can't usually smell anything else either! They're very effective, but I would recommend building up to their use. It's unrealistic to expect your body, which is possibly chockful of synthetic toxins, to be able to make the switch instantly. It may take a few days for the toxic residues to be eliminated, and then you'll see if the mineral deodorant works for you.

Another great tip is to wash your crystal deodorant and use it on spots if they appear (sadly, even at my ripe old age I seem to get the occasional zit). You simply rub gently across the spot and, as if by magic, it seems to dry it up quickly. They're incredibly good value at around £3 – £6 for the natural deodorant, which could last up to a year and a half if you look after it. If you prefer a spray deodorant, most companies now offer one fragranced with essential oils or with organic plant extracts to help combat odours.

Stockists include:

- www.weleda.co.uk
- www.faithinnature.com
- www.pitrok.co.uk
- www.greenpeople.co.uk

Yet again, you can also make your own – see the recipes section (page 50).

Stainless Steel

I'm sure you've come across stainless steel bars to help neutralize odours. They're often sold to rub your hands on after chopping garlic, etc., but you can also now buy the amazing body stick which looks like a roll-on deodorant but is simply a stick of stainless steel. Now please don't ask me how this works, but astonishingly it seems to! Available from www.thenaturalcollection.com.

SUNSCREENS
I've written extensively on this before, and in truth I feel I'm still learning as the parameters keep changing. You'll hear a huge amount of conflicting advice about the use of sunscreens and the serious effects of being sunburnt; all I can do is add my two-penn'orth. First (and perhaps rather controversially) I believe we are nation overly obsessed with sunscreens. We wear moisturizing creams with an SPF factor even on cold winter days, for heaven's sake! I believe it's vital for us to get some exposure to the sun, in moderation. Many years ago heliotherapy was popular and proved beneficial for many conditions. Patients were encouraged to literally sun-bathe under controlled conditions. See the excellent book by Richard Hobday: *Healing Sun*.

Of course, with climate change and the concerns over the ozone layer I am not about to encourage girlfriends to don a bikini and veg out while the sun beats down for hours, but I do think that 15 to 30 minutes a day is essential.

Vitamin D
Surveys have shown recently that there are increased numbers of people with vitamin D deficiency. Adequate levels of vitamin D are essential and can even reduce your cancer risk. In fact, according to Dr Michael F. Holick of the Boston University School of Medicine, there would be 25 per cent fewer fatalities from breast cancer if women took

adequate levels of vitamin D. I'm sure these deficiencies are partly due to our obsession with plastering ourselves with sunscreen so that the beneficial UVA rays can't penetrate. (It's the UV*B* rays that can be harmful.)

For the times when you need to be out in the sun, the trick is to be out and about but not to sunbathe – stay active. You'll know how much sun your skin type can tolerate. Personally I am very sensitive and burn at the first sniff of a UVB ray, so for me the best sunscreen is protective clothing. I call it going for the film star image – I wear huge pashminas or thin shawls, huge sunglasses, a big floppy hat and always sit or walk in the shade. If you use natural mineral make-up (or decide to after reading what I have to say about it later on!), you'll find that many of the foundations contain titanium dioxide. This natural mineral is an effective blocker of both UVA and UVB rays, giving you the added bonus of 'inbuilt' sun protection. Shea butter, sesame oil and jojoba oil have natural SPFs of 4–6.

Some organic oils and butters have a naturally low SPF with high moisturizing and skin-repairing ability, too.

Natural Suncreams

If your work (or your life) requires you to be exposed to the sun for longer than 30 minutes a day, choose the most natural suncream you can find. Sadly, most commercial suncreams contain a hair-raising number of potentially toxic ingredients including chemicals which generate free radicals (proven carcinogens) and many other ingredients which have been linked to hormone disruption, allergies, skin sensitivity and rashes. It's best to opt for a sunblock that creates a physical barrier, which aims to reflect the UV rays.

Of course, the problem is that these tend to be opaque and white – which is fine for a diamond shape across a surfer's or skier's nose, but most people don't want to have that all over their bodies on a daily basis.

Zinc oxide is probably the safest of these, but beware of companies who now offer it as a transparent sunblock, as it often contains nano-particles which are thought to be extremely harmful depending on their size. Nanotechnology uses penetration-enhancing ingredients that bypass the skin's protective barrier and pass more deeply into the body and bloodstream.

SPF

The whole SPF factor thing is confusing, too. We tend to think the higher number, the better it is – but in fact a sunscreen with an SPF factor of 30 gives only about 2 per cent more protection than SPF 20.

Some of my favourite natural sunscreens include those from:

- www.greenpeople.co.uk
- www.weleda.co.uk
- www.yaoh.co.uk
- www.drhauschka.co.uk

After-sun Care

One of the best ways to cool your body after you've been in the sun is to apply coconut oil or vitamin E oil. If you're unlucky enough to get actual sunburn, then use aloe vera gel (straight from the plant is best; failing that, try the Pure and Natural Aloe Vera Gel from Pure Nuff Stuff: www.purenuffstuff.co.uk).

INSECT REPELLENTS

What you need to ask yourself, is what is in the insect repellent sprays or creams that really work? Answer: fairly scary chemicals, including, in many incidences, pesticides such as DEET, which has been linked to a huge range of health issues. Children are very susceptible to its effects.

It's often said that you can boost your body's natural defences by ensuring you have adequate levels of vitamin B, because it's thought that insects (particularly mosquitoes) don't favour people who clearly have enough of this important vitamin. In the name of honesty I must tell you I dosed up liberally on vitamin B but still ended up badly bitten on a recent trip to Turkey, but by all means try it! I can't help but think perhaps I am just particularly attractive to bugs and beasties – not the desired outcome of all this effort into natural beauty, but hey ho!

It's thought that eating garlic will put off insects, too (but then you have to weigh up whether it mightn't also put off highly desirable guys!).

There are some natural repellents now, including Neem oil-based ones which seem to work. I also have an excellent spray called Bugs at Bay from www.homescents.co.uk which contains essential oils and so far has worked for me.

You might want to try making your own anti-bug spray by adding a few drops of rosemary, citronella, eucalyptus and lavender to a small amount of mineral water. If it doesn't put off bugs, at least it will smell great!

You can also get Don't Bite Me patches (try repellant patches from www.dontbitemepatch.com) and 100 per cent organic balms such as the anti-bug balm from Badger Balm in most good pharmacies. I've also tried applying neat tea tree oil which seems effective. I'd love to hear what works for you.

FACE UP

So, we've dealt with the body beautiful – but what about the girlfriend's face? 'I'm NOT ditching my moisturizer or make-up,' I hear you cry. Please bear with me.

For starters, have a sneak preview of the Food chapter: if you eat for optimum health, your skin will look brighter and healthier and fine lines will be reduced far more noticeably than any conventional moisture cream will achieve.

If you've never tried face oils before, let me persuade you to try them. When I was younger and had greasy skin, I was convinced 'oil upon oil' would be a disaster. To my surprise, however, I found that a tiny amount made all the problems I'd had over the years disappear. I now recommend everyone give facial oils a try. Most people find that oils regulate their pores where creams can sometimes aggravate.

This could be because rich protective creams take a long time to be absorbed by the skin. They are designed to shield the skin from the elements. Too much hydration, though (which can happen if we ladle on the creams), the skin becomes a bit lazy and doesn't produce as much sebum. So it feels dry, we reapply cream, and the end result is precisely the sagging, drooping look we were trying to avoid!

The ideal is to nourish the skin's layers, and then protect. Oils nourish but don't put any water in, and because there is no water, this removes the need for a preservative – the very ingredient that can prove most tricky to replicate with natural sources.

Vegetable oils restore what I'm assured is called the 'hydro-lipidic film' of the skin.

All I know is that my skin is better than it has ever been, now that I use facial oils.

Girlfriends' Natural Secrets ... Once a week loofah your face. Gentle circular motions preferably with a gentle body wash. You can buy small round loofahs for the face. A gentle exfoliant will give you a clear and smooth complexion, and also removes all the dead skin.

Take make-up off (including waterproof mascara) with damp cotton wool soaked in almond oil. ALWAYS take your make-up off at night; if you find yourself not at home, olive oil, sunflower oil or any good oil will do.'

– Rosi Flood, Costume designer

Best Facial Oils

If you want to buy facial oils there are some excellent ones; they last for ages so don't be put off by a seemingly high price, you need only a tiny amount. Look at facial oils from:

- www.inlight-online.co.uk
- www.forestsecretsskincare.com
- www.herbfarmacy.co.uk
- www.lucyrussellorganics.co.uk
- www.annemarieborlind.co.uk
- www.greenpeople.co.uk

Going DIY

This is one area, though, where it's very simple, cheap and effective to go DIY.

In truth any oil will do. Virgin olive oil works well, though it can be a little heavy. Apricot kernel or jojoba oils also work well. You can combine your chosen oil with a little salt, too, to turn your facial treatment into a more exfoliating scrub. See the recipes beginning on page 38.

Facial Masks and Scrubs

Once you're making fresh juices regularly (and if not, why not?!), you'll be delighted to know that not all of the fruit pulp needs to be discarded. If you make a healthy green veggie juice, for example, the pulp will contain amazing live enzymes which you can apply to sore skin and watch it heal. Cucumber contains many vitamins and minerals including folic acid, and is highly diuretic (removes water) so it's great for cleansing the skin and excellent for your hair, too. Pineapple is high in potassium as well as vitamin C and folic acid, and it cleanses the intestines and boosts the immune system, to name just two of the benefits. Pretty much any fresh fruit or veg makes a nice face pack!

Girlfriends' Natural Secrets ... Top tip (given to me by my granny!): When slicing a cucumber, use the end bits as an instant face freshener – just smooth the cut side over the skin for a lovely fresh feel. Tightens the pores, too!
  – Liz Scambler, director, www.teamlollipop.co.uk

Make-up

This is one area where the natural alternative options have really grown. When I wrote my first book there were only one or two ranges, but now there's a wealth of choice. Even if you're new to natural skincare and beauty, you will, I'm sure, recognize that regular cosmetics usually contain a fair amount of complicated chemicals and potentially toxic ingredients. We've all seen the scaremongering tales that do the rounds on the internet about lead being in many lipsticks and people who have had terrible allergic reactions or problems with their eyesight due to mascaras (often way past their sell-by date and which have therefore become toxic over time).

More and more synthetic ingredients have been added to cosmetics over the years, probably because it makes them cheaper to manufacture and of course extends their shelf-life, but at what price to our health and well-being? As with all skincare and household products, the tiny amount in each product item is not enough to cause any problem, but the cumulative effect over years of use can certainly affect us, especially with lipsticks, which are quickly ingested. It's thought that at least 10 per cent of the chemicals licensed for use in cosmetics may not have been tested on humans, so it makes great sense to opt for natural ranges that don't contain parabens, preservatives, synthetic dyes or colours, petrochemicals or bismuth oxychloride.

The good news – and you knew I'd have some – is that you can now buy a natural version of every make-up product, even those much adored and best-selling light-reflective concealers!

Foundation

Mineral powders have become all the rage now for foundation. It's a very different approach to using cream bases or even pressed powder compacts, but they do give a good coverage even for acne, while still looking very fresh and fairly flawless if applied correctly. The trick is to shake a tiny bit of mineral powder into the lid and, using a nice full brush, circle it around a little on the lid before applying in big circular movements to your face and neck.

Some companies offer a foundation which is a concealer, foundation and a powder in one. The great thing is they don't clog the pores or irritate the skin, and many have the added benefit of increased natural sun protection.

Natural mineral powders are made from natural pigments and oxides and, because mineral powders are inorganic and contain no moisture, bacteria won't grow, therefore preservatives don't need to be added.

Concealers and Blushers
You can also get powder 'concealers' and gorgeous blushers. I've also used an excellent concealer pencil which works well, and a light cream which is best applied with a small brush.

Eyes
There are many vibrant powder eyeshadows to choose from, including great sparkly ones. Again, the trick is not to get too much on the brush or it flies everywhere, messing up your foundation so that then that needs to be reapplied!

You can also get natural versions of eyeliner, mascara, lipstick, the works.

My favourite ranges are:

- www.inikacosmetics.co.uk
- www.lilylolo.co.uk
- www.lavera.co.uk
- www.elysambre.nat-cos.com
- www.greenpeople.co.uk
- www.puritycosmetics.co.uk

Girlfriends' Natural Secrets ... Cheap, effective and works for me – I use hemp oil for a cleanser and diluted rose water and few drops of tea tree oil for a toner.

At the first signs of cold/flu (or even general unwell feelings) copious amounts of lemon, manuka honey and fresh ginger drink, and rubbed garlic on toast or garlic butter to have on anything (or put in soup, on veg) – use any way to get raw garlic into you!

Favourite herbs – lemon balm for pain (particularly period pains), rosemary for tension headache, valerian for sleep, nettle for skin.

Girlfriends' Aspiration ... Happiness, it keeps you young, and one day before I get too old to do the hippie trail!
– Patchouli www.hippie-trail.com

Teenage Skin

Most teenagers don't want to be seen using mum's skin-care ranges. A few natural companies have recognized the need for affordable natural skincare for teenagers that comes in funky packaging. Try the Oy range from www.greenpeople.co.uk, which includes the excellent Cover and Clear Spot It (a tinted moisturizer that acts as an antibacterial spot treatment) and the handmade skincare range from www.naturalcollateral.com.

WATER

If we want great skin we need to drink copious amounts of water (more about this in the Food chapter), but when it comes to the water we wash with, believe it or not our household water could mean serious skin conditions even if we are using the best, most natural skincare products and make-up in the world.

To start with, many people simply wash too often. You may be reeling back in horror at that statement, but it really is true.

The Hazards of Chlorine

Washing in heavily chlorinated water is very drying for your skin. Chlorine is used worldwide for its disinfecting power, and is added to our water to protect us from water-borne infections – and it can also be responsible for some fairly adverse effects on our skin and hair. Chlorine can destroy much-needed proteins in our bodies. Depleted of protein, skin and hair can become very dry and unmanageable. Chlorine also strips the natural protective oils from skin and hair, causing excess dryness. After clinical studies were carried out for over a year at the Department of Dermatology, Toyama Medical and Pharmaceutical University in Japan, the researchers stated that residual chlorine in bathing water reduces the water-holding capacity of the top layer of our skin, which results in the skin drying out more easily, compromising the skin's barrier and potentially leading to infections and irritation.

Even at very low levels, chlorine causes damage to skin and hair. And half of our daily chlorine exposure is from showering, so the water you shower in should be a priority, particularly if you suffer from sensitive or delicate skin prone to dryness, eczema, psoriasis or any chemical sensitivities.

The great news is you can buy a shower filter to remove the chlorine and soften the bathing water. It fits easily onto most shower units between the shower head and hose, or there's a ball that hangs under the taps to dechlorinate the bathwater as it runs.

If you're interested in the technical data, the dechlorination filters are made up of KDF, which removes the chlorine and bacteria plus heavy metals and pollutants. I have a shower filter and it has lasted for a year. It's advised that they last 6 to 12 months depending on frequency of use, but the good thing is it's clear so you can see that when the golden section of the filtration unit turns a black/greenish colour it will need to be replaced. For the dechlorination ball it's not so obvious when you'll need to replace it, but I'd aim for around every 12 months. The dechlorination ball is just under £50 and the shower filter is around £35 from Sensitive Skincare Company www.sensitiveskincareco.com or www.janeysnaturalstore.com.

DIY BEAUTY

It's so easy and feels so rewarding to create your own personalized, handmade, natural skincare – and no, I don't mean toiling over a double boiler for hours. My recipes are quick and easy and cost next to nothing. You'll find most of the ingredients you need already in your kitchen cupboard. A few to get you started include:

- Oatmeal – It's healing and soothing for sensitive skin. You can grind it to make it finer.
- Cornflour – Good for oily skin
- Ground almonds – Gently exfoliating while providing oils for the skin

- Sugar and salt – Any type but coarse is best, opt for Himalayan salt or Dead Sea salt, great to add to olive oil to make a scrub or exfoliant
- Used coffee grounds – Antibacterial, exfoliating and stimulating, great for cellulite

Ayurvedic recipes often use ground sunflower seeds, ground oats, brewer's yeast and various other 'foodstuffs' such as chickpea flour and lentils. Almost anything, if it's good for you to eat, will be beneficial for your skin! (Cooked foods notwithstanding!)

Herbs and Flowers

What's out and about in your garden (or in a nearby meadow!) is also great to add to your beauty regime. Dried marigold flowers, dandelion leaves, sprigs of lavender and fresh herbs such as parsley and rosemary can all be used. Moisten the dried ingredients with:

- Coconut oil – It has so many uses, but remember it solidifies in cold temperatures.
- Cacao butter – Also fantastic but will need to be melted before use.
- Olive oil – Soothing, moisturizing and contains antioxidants which help protect the skin from the effects of ageing. You can use it for both cleansing and moisturizing.
- Other lighter oils are great to use as a base for aromatherapy massage oils, facial oils and scrubs. Try sweet almond oil, jojoba, carrot oil, avocado oil or wheatgerm oil.
- Essential oils, of course – Choose from geranium, rose, lemon or tea tree oil, to name just a few of my favourites.

- Citrus oils – Lime juice, lemon juice and orange juice will add an astringent to your mix, which is great for oily skins and will give added vitamin C.
- Honey – So long as you're not vegan, of course, honey is great because it's antibacterial, soothing and healing. If you can afford it, manuka honey is incredibly effective at treating minor wounds. For more information try googling 'apitherapy' – you'll be amazed at its uses.
- Floral waters – Lavender water is excellent. Pure rosewater makes a wonderful toner. Worth sourcing from aromatherapy suppliers because some floral waters sold in pharmacies contain artificial ingredients.
- Live yoghurt – Contains lactic acid and is very cooling. Adds a creamy quality to homemade cleansers. You can also use milk.
- Cucumber – Peeled and puréed, this is very cooling and good as a toner. Also, cucumber slices help revive tired skin and eyes.
- Aloe vera gel or juice – Very useful. Of course you can snip the juice from an aloe vera plant, too – perfect for healing wounds or minor burns.
- Avocado – Rich in antioxidants and good for dry skin. Any fruits are good, of course. Mashed bananas always feel soothing and you can use grated lemon and orange peel, too.
- Fruit juices – Fresh apple juice is great for exfoliating. Tomato juice is rich in antioxidants. In fact, any freshly extracted juice is fantastic and, as already mentioned, you can use the pulp from fresh juices to concoct a great face mask.
- Beeswax – This is also worth getting hold of; you can

melt it easily and use for lipbalms or rich hand creams. You can buy beeswax from local beekeepers or at farmers' markets.

Girlfriends' Natural Secrets ... Once a week I fill a small bowl with raw cane sugar and a teaspoon of oil (almond, olive, or whatever is to hand), mix it together and rub the mixture all over my hands in a washing motion for about 5 minutes. Then rinse off in warm water. So simple. It's great for feet, too, and I've used a larger quantity as an all-over-body exfoliation.

Girlfriends' Aspirations ... As well as keeping young and gorgeous!!! I am really fond of keeping the romance alive, and for our next wedding anniversary (six months away) I would love to sing my husband a song. I'm taking secret guitar lessons (ssshh). He's going to be so shocked and surprised – it's going to be amazing seeing his face.

– Heather Bestel www.heatherbestel.com

Before I give you some very simple recipes, let me tell you about my ayurvedic pampering experience.

Ayurvedic Beauty

I first came to experience a little bit about Ayurvedic medicine when I was pregnant. A wonderful Indian birth guru prescribed various Ayurvedic herbs. I also had some incredibly healing Ayurvedic massages, and was given lots of advice about how to use the most natural ingredients for skincare and beauty.

Ayurveda developed in India over 5,000 years ago. Some say it's the world's most complete and integrated system of healing. The word *Ayurveda* translates as 'Life knowledge', and it can indeed teach us to acknowledge our own individual constitution and how to create balance in our lives. It uses a holistic mix of diet, detoxification and purification techniques, yoga, breathing exercises, herbal and mineral remedies, meditation and massage therapy.

The website www.kalyanatherapies.co.uk offers an excellent explanation of Ayurveda therapy:

> *'The whole universe consists of the five elements:* **space, air, fire, water** *and* **earth**. *Every disease is an imbalance of these elements and Ayurveda therapy is targeted at its root cause using meditation, massage, exercise, medication and nutrition. It places a strong emphasis on preventative measures to* **feel better, look better** *and* **have more energy** *in old age.'*

The experts at this website can offer an analysis of your constitution to determine which energy is dominant in your body at this present moment. According to Ayurveda, a person's constitution is the balance of three *doshas* – biological forces that govern the body. So, for example, some people love spicy hot foods while others prefer cooling foods, some of us thrive as vegetarians while some need meat. The three basic types are:

1. *Vata* – People who tend to be of low body weight and feel the cold easily, often with dry skin.

2. *Pitta* – Usually hot, often medium build and with oily skin that's prone to rashes.
3. *Kapha* – Often heavy or stocky, with thick wavy hair and pale skin.

At my recent pampering session, I had a mini-consultation and learned that I was definitely Pitta in constitution. The Ayurvedic practitioner then recommended the best natural ingredients for my skin type and gave me a wonderful mini-facial with homespun goodies. We started with:

Aloe Vera Cleanser
– 30 ml aloe vera gel (you can buy it or snip directly from the plant)
– 30 ml rosewater
– 50 ml olive oil
– 4 drops rose essential oil
– 2 drops grapefruit seed extract

It felt very cooling to my pitta skin! Then came:

Walnut, Lentil and Chickpea Scrub
– Equal amounts (a few tablespoons each) cooked green lentils, finely ground walnuts and chickpea flour
– 1 tablespoon honey
– 1 tablespoon rosewater
– Enough yoghurt to make a paste

This felt a bit moist and sloppy to apply but smelt gorgeous.

After a quick facial steam with mint, lemon balm and calendula leaves in the water, we applied:

Cucumber Mask
- A few teaspoons brewer's yeast
- A few teaspoons finely powdered oats
- Chunk of peeled liquidized cucumber
- 2 tablespoons plain yoghurt
- 1 teaspoon runny honey
- 1 drop essential oil

Whizz all ingredients together in a high-speed blender.

As I lay relaxing with my mask on, the therapist laid thin slices of cucumber over my face and eyes. It felt extremely cooling!

After washing off the mask – which felt rather like removing green porridge – I used a pure rosewater toner, then the therapist used a thick moisturizer with geranium and apricot oils. That one was a bridge too far for busy old me, requiring adding emulsifying wax to a rose petal infusion – but there are much simpler moisturizers that will do the job just as well. Here's one that is meant for *Vata* skin types but is gorgeous for everyone.

Rich Rose Cream
- 7 g beeswax
- 2 tablespoons almond oil
- 30 ml rosewater
- 4 drops rose oil

Melt together the beeswax and almond oil. Remove the bowl from the heat and slowly add the rosewater, stirring constantly. Keep stirring as it starts to cool and add the rose oil. Stir until the mixture thickens and then transfer to a sterilized jar.

- For more on Ayurvedic beauty and for a consultation see www.kalyanatherapies.co.uk

CREATE YOUR OWN SKINCARE

Here are a few simple ideas to get you started. You'll soon realize that it's easy-peasy to replace the suggested ingredients with whatever you have lying around.

It's usually best just to make enough to use straight away; if you do make more and want to keep for use later, then remember if no preservatives are added you will need to store in an airtight container and usually in the fridge. Treat handmade natural skincare as you would fresh foods without preservatives.

Make-up Remover

Good old olive oil works a treat as an emergency cleanser and eye make-up remover. It could be a little heavy for use twice daily, though.

I don't wear eye make-up every day so I find that, when I do, a tiny amount of almond oil on a cotton pad works well. (It's lighter than olive oil.)

Cleansing cloths are also great. Try the equivalent of a microfibre cloth for use in the kitchen, they're made in the form of a glove, so great for removing make-up. You can also buy an organic cotton facecloth from www.sensitiveskincareco.com.

Cleansing Wash

The simplest cleansing wash can be made using Castile liquid soap:

- 50 ml Castile liquid soap
- 10 drops pure essential oil of your choice

Shake it all up and it's ready to use. It will store for a while, too, if you wanted to increase the quantities. You can also add almond oil (about 5 ml) for dry skin.

Girlfriends' Natural Secrets ... I try to remember that oil is good at dissolving oil and dirt from the skin. I use almond oil as a cleanser every day on my oily skin. I smooth a 50p size amount all over my face, making sure I massage it in, and then use a muslin cloth dampened with warm water to remove. This removes make-up, including mascara, as it doesn't hurt your eyes, and leaves you with wonderful clean skin which is also soft but not greasy. Over time it also decreases the amount of oil your skin produces, as the skin isn't constantly being stripped and trying to overcompensate by producing more.

– Mel Horrod

Toner or Skin Spritzer

Toners will remove any make-up traces, refresh the skin and work as an astringent to balance the skin's own pH level.

For normal or combination skin, try fresh cucumber juice (peel the cucumber first).

For oily skin, diluted lemon juice is brilliant. I also sometimes use cooled chamomile tea which feels really refreshing.

Another simple toner is just pure floral water. You can buy these from good aromatherapy suppliers (www.potions.co.uk or www.tortuerouge.co.uk). Rosewater is probably the easiest and most obvious; you can also add witch hazel – my menopausal girlfriend keeps a little spritzer bottle of rosewater and witch hazel 50/50 in her handbag at all times and sprays her face and neck at the first sign of a hot flush.

You can add herbal infusions, tinctures or teas to floral waters. Use your own herbs if you have green fingers, or buy dried herbs such as chamomile, fennel, elderflower, lemon-balm, etc. (there is a wealth of choice) or even use a herbal tea bag. Green tea especially is rich in antioxidants and is thought to be anti-ageing.

You can also use vinegars such as apple cider vinegar (which is also a fantastic hair rinse). Of course it's easy to make your own herbal vinegars, too, by adding chopped herbs or flowers to a jar of apple cider vinegar, leaving in a warm place for a couple of weeks (shaking the bottle a couple of times a day) and then straining off the vinegar.

Lavender and myrrh work well together (yes, myrrh of wise men fame) and offer a healing antiseptic toner for oily or blemished skin:

- 100 ml lavender water
- 10 drops myrrh essential oil

Honey is very healing, too:

- 1 tsp honey
- 100 ml warm water
- 2 drops bergamot essential oil

Dissolve the honey in the warm water, then add the bergamot oil. This one will need to be kept in the fridge.

The possibilities really are endless, so enjoy making your own aromatic mists!

Moisturizers

Moisturizers help to keep your skin soft and add moisture to the surface layer of the skin, so if you're going to make a cream it will need to have added water. This then means you will need to add a preservative and usually some kind of emulsifier to hold the water and oil together. When you apply creams, use a tiny spatula to take a small amount from the jar rather than putting your fingers in there each time, which could result in bacteria forming.

There are lots of recipes for great moisturizers if you don't mind getting involved in heating and melting shea butters, adding emulsifying waxes, etc. For some excellent recipes see *The Ultimate Natural Beauty Book* by Josephine Fairley or *The Holistic Beauty Book* by Star Khechara.

For now, though, I want to offer you only the quickest, simplest options, so I'd suggest making a gel-based moisturizer using organic aloe vera gel. This can be used on its own; it makes a great moisturizer and, interestingly, is great as a shaving lotion for your fella, too!

- 100 ml aloe vera gel
- 5 drops almond oil
- 10 drops essential oil

Simply mix together the aloe vera gel and the almond oil, then add the essential oil. Rose otto essential oil makes a particularly good anti-ageing moisturizing gel. Lavender also works well with aloe vera. There's no reason why you can't experiment and add two or three different aromas.

Essential Oils

I've already indicated that in my opinion facial oils are the best treatment for all skin types. They will help to hydrate the skin, balance the production of sebum and are great at fighting infection. The other great benefit is that, as I've already made clear, they can be absorbed into the skin and have further therapeutic benefits. They also smell great and increase your happiness levels! (See the chapter on The Power of Fragrance!).

There are so many essential oils to choose from. Initially I asked a qualified aromatherapist to make me up a facial oil recipe using exactly the right oils that she felt I needed at that time (I was feeling very stressed and had a cold coming on). As time went on I became more confident and experimented with making my own blends.

The most important thing to remember is that you must dilute the essential oils in a base or carrier oil (lavender oil and tea tree oil are the exceptions as they can be applied neat – in fact they work great to treat spots!). It's also important to remember that certain aromatherapy oils can cause irritation. Some people can be sensitive or allergic, so treat oils with caution. Always consult a practitioner before you use essential oils if you are pregnant, particularly the first three months. Avoid certain oils if you have high blood pressure, too.

Girlfriends' Natural Secrets ... Tea tree oil is great for nails. Soak fingers and toes in warm water and tea tree oil for 10 minutes once a fortnight to stop them getting brittle.

Nettle products are good for everything! Nettle root powder, nettle tea, nettle juice, etc.

– Amy Trotter, administrator, Yestolife
– alternatives for people with cancer
www.yestolife.org.uk

There are too many essential oils to list here, but I find a great reference book is *The Fragrant Pharmacy* by Valerie Ann Worwood.

Make sure you source oils from a good supplier. Always buy pure essential oils, not 'fragrance' oils or blends.

Essential oils and skincare can be bought from www.tortuerouge.co.uk, www.justaromatherapy.co.uk, www.essentialoilcompany.com and www.potions.co.uk.

Oil blends do have their place, just not as facial oils. They are wonderfully therapeutic for lifting your spirits, not for applying topically but great to have around. Children especially benefit from them. One company called *Special Little People* (www.speciallittlepeople.co.uk) has created lovely blends to help children with confidence, exams, sleeping, etc. The box contains a tiny handkerchief to sniff the oil from.

To lift your spirits while travelling, try an aromatherapy bracelet from Aroma Angel www.wristangel.co.uk.

Girlfriends' Natural Secrets ... *At the first signs of a zit, dab neat echinacea tincture onto the spot and prepare to be amazed. I also add a few drops to a little of my usual face oil if a patch of skin could do with a healing boost. It's great for helping scars to disappear.*

Girlfriends' Aspirations ... *I'd write comedy, every day – is there anything better than hearing people laugh?*
– Petre Sefton www.tortuerouge.com
(and host of natural perfume courses in France)

Creating Your Own Facial Oil

Choose a base oil which is fairly light and easily absorbed. I've already mentioned coconut oil; it's possible to use coconut oil and olive oil on the face, but for facial oils with added essential oils it's better to choose one such as jojoba, sweet almond, apricot kernel, evening primrose or rosehip oil. Depending on how sensitive your skin is, you can add up to 25 drops of essential oil to 100 ml carrier oil, but it's a good idea to start with a maximum of 10 drops.

A few suggestions:

Combination Skin Healing Oil
- 100 ml almond oil
- 5 drops lavender oil
- 2 drops frankincense
- 2 drops manuka
- 1 drop german chamomile oil

Oily Skin Healing Oil
- 50 ml carrot oil mixed with 50 ml wheatgerm oil
- 5 drops lavender oil
- 2 drops rose oil
- 2 drops geranium oil

Anti-ageing Oil
- 50 ml rosehip mixed with 50 ml sweet almond oil
- 2 drops lavender oil
- 2 drops rose oil
- 1 drop frankincense

Girlfriends' Natural Secrets ... *Having lived up a mountain in southwestern Turkey for eight or nine months of each year for the last six years, with not a* shop or healthstore in sight, I have had to become more resourceful. My natural beauty discovery and secret is olive oil sourced locally from my village and from a few olive trees around our house. It is not just for eating, but has become a multi-purpose natural ingredient that I use daily with really good results.

I use it as a hair treatment, on my hands, as a body moisturizer, for massaging feet and heels. For a foot bath, I add 2 tablespoons of olive oil to a bowl of hot water and soak my feet for 15 minutes. I also use it as a base oil, adding 3–5 drops of pure essential lavender oil.

– Miriam Mcquirk, writer

Exfoliators, Scrubs and Masks

Basic Exfoliating Scrub

– Mix oatmeal and water to slough off dead skin.

You can also use cornflour, especially if your skin is oily.

Add honey to form an exfoliating paste. Yoghurt will make it creamy.

Face Mask for Oily Skin

– 2 teaspoons cornflour
– 1 egg white

Mix and apply, then wash off after 15 minutes.

Pore-cleansing Coconut Oil Exfoliant

– 3 teaspoons coconut oil
– 1 tablespoon yoghurt
– 1 tablespoon Dead Sea salt or Himalayan salt

Mix to a paste, apply and rinse off with water.

Dead Sea Salt Scrub
- 2 tablespoons Dead Sea salt
- 2 tablespoons almond oil
- 1 teaspoon lemon juice

If you have normal skin you can replace the lemon with a drop of tea tree oil or a teaspoon of honey.

Face and Body Masks
Almost any foodie bits will work as a mask, it's just a case of combining ingredients and experimenting with what feels nice.

Honey, Jojoba, Yoghurt Soothing Mask
- 2 tablespoons yoghurt
- 1 teaspoon of jojoba
- 1 tablespoon honey

Apply to face, leave on till the yoghurt dries, then wash off with warm water.

Fruity Cooling Mask
- Half an avocado
- Half a pear
- Half a banana
- A few drops of lemon juice
- A tiny amount of cream cheese to bind.

This one is good if the ingredients are mixed together in a blender.

Chocolate Face Mask
- 2 tablespoons raw organic cocoa powder
- 1 tablespoon honey
- 1 tablespoon yoghurt
- 3 teaspoons fine oatmeal

Blend together the ingredients, apply and leave on for 20 minutes.

If you'd prefer the mask to be moisturizing but not exfoliating, then leave out the oatmeal.

Of course you can increase quantities and add coconut oil for a full body wrap – a fantastic way of having all the benefits of chocolate without any calories!

Girlfriends' Natural Secrets ... When I have finished eating an avocado, I like to scoop out the last bits from the skin and rub into my hands and face – sooo creamy.

One thing I like is to mash up an avocado, mix in 1 drop geranium oil and a sprinkling of pink salt and massage all over my body for a natural scrub (and it doesn't matter if a bit falls in my mouth!).

Girlfriends' Aspirations ... My aspiration is simply to just sing on Jools Holland – I love him and his show! I am determined! Oh, and perform live on stage with Eminem – my little brother would be so proud!!!

– Victoria Leith, www.freshandlivemama.com

Lip Balm

I'm not a fan of regular lip balms or lip salves; most contain petroleum or mineral oils and actually result in drying out the sensitive lip area rather than softening or protecting it. Fortunately you can buy natural lip balms or make your own. Sadly, to do this you do need to do a bit of 'melting' with the base ingredients. Beeswax, for example, needs to be melted to exactly the right consistency, but here's the simplest recipe I've tried.

Shea Butter Lip Balm
- 1 tablespoon shea butter
- Honey

Melt the shea butter in a bowl over hot water. Stir in a tiny amount of honey. Put it into a clean 15-ml pot, leave it to cool and put in the fridge to set.

You can also add pure essential oils to lip balms. 1 drop of peppermint or spearmint tastes great and has antiseptic properties.

Deodorants

I've already stressed that it's never a good idea to use an antiperspirant, and remember that any natural deodorants won't stop you perspiring but they *will* stop the unsavoury smell.

Simple Homemade Deodorant
- 50 ml almond or jojoba oil
- 6 drops bergamot essential oil

You may prefer to replace the bergamot with another citrus oil such as neroli, lemon, mandarin or lime.

Be careful not to expose your armpits to direct sunlight, though, as the oils are photo-sensitive!

If you prefer a deodorant stick:

Get a discarded 100 ml deodorant case or similar.

Stand a glass jar in boiling water. Add:

- 1½ tablespoons beeswax
- ½ tablespoon cocoa butter
- 1 tablespoon coconut oil

Once those have melted, stir in:

- 15 drops rosemary essential oil
- 25 drops lavender essential oil
- 3 drops jojoba oil

Pour the mixture into the deodorant case, leave to cool and set. Even easier is to make a paste by adding a few drops of water to a little bicarbonate of soda – apply and leave!

Another strange one is that you can rub a little lemon juice under your armpit. Yes, it's effective, but keep away from wasps!

Girlfriends' Natural Secrets ... Sweating is one of the body's essential functions, eliminating toxins through the skin, for a clear complexion steam your face weekly – a fantastic method of deep cleansing the skin. I fill a bowl with boiling water and add a few sage leaves, cover my head with a towel and try to stay like that for up to 15 minutes. Then I splash my face with cold water. Refreshed!

– Abigail James, organic therapist
www.abigailjames.com

Janey's Guide to Beautiful Hair, Teeth and Nails

On every talk I do across the UK, there's one question that always comes up: how can I colour my hair naturally? Answer: sadly, unless your hair is in the red spectrum and you can use henna, there's nothing that actually 'falls off a tree' – but this is where my sometimes 'imperfect' approach comes in. If you're lucky enough to have never coloured your hair, then leave well alone, but for most of us that's not our reality.

I recommend that you try and locate a salon not too far from you that uses organic and mineral colours. Even then, don't get too excited: most of these preparations still include some synthetic chemicals – but they're definitely more gentle on hair than the usual harsh colourings we're used to.

Daniel Field is the pioneer of organic and mineral hairdressing. I am lucky and local enough to be able to visit his salon in Herts, where he uses seaweed lightener on my blonde hair.

Another great salon using organic and mineral products is Spirit Organic in the Cotswolds (www.spiritorganic.com).

There are two branches: one in Stow and one in Broadway. The founder, Tabitha James Kraan, has a wonderfully refreshing approach to natural hair care – it's not often I find a hairdresser who agrees with my stance on not washing your hair too often.

SHAMPOOING

Tabitha has written this for us:

'I believe that these days we all wash our hair too often. We are therefore literally washing the life out of our hair! We use shampoos which are too strong and that over-stimulate the sebaceous glands, creating an over-oily scalp. This leaves the scalp and hair feeling like it needs to be washed again and therefore keeps up this repetitive cycle of daily washing. The complaints I hear and see for myself most often are of greasy roots and dry ends, frizzy hair, dehydrated fluffy hair, lifeless hair that lacks lustre and hair that HAS to be washed daily.

'My advice would be invest in the mildest, most organic shampoo you can find to fit your budget. Bear in mind that it will last because you won't be using it every day.

'Expect it not to froth. Lather is actually a problem for hair because it over-chelates the hair (which leaves the cuticle open and the hair more tangly).

'Think about washing your scalp and the root area of the hair, and never encourage foam through the length of the hair; when you rinse that will be enough to refresh the hair.

'Then you need to assess whether the hair needs a conditioner, detangler or just some oil.'

Homemade Conditioning Treatment
Avocado (mashed) with extra virgin olive oil

'Work through the length of the hair, leave for about 20 minutes in cling film and a towel, then shampoo out.

'I would recommend that the ideal washing routine should be once a week. If you are currently washing every day you will need to retrain your scalp gradually. First wash every other day, then every two days, etc., allowing around four weeks between each change to allow your scalp to settle down.

'You can use other products to help get you through this period. Dry shampoo is excellent but usually very chemical. Try a natural body powder instead; Dr Hauschka do a great silk body powder and it works really well as a dry shampoo. Just apply to the roots, massage in and then give the hair a good brush, then dress into shape. Fantastic for big hair, too.

'You can also just rinse your hair with water and blow it dry or let it dry naturally. Naturally curly hair can be rinsed and conditioned but not shampooed.'

Using Heat on Your Hair
'I would encourage a respectful use of heat on the hair. Heat can do a lot of damage if overdone, and should therefore be used sparingly.

'There are great styling products on the market that work in harmony with the hair and give your blow dry or set

*extra life. I love John Masters Organics Sweet Orange &
Silk Protein Organic Styling Gel.*

*'The right product will give you heat protection and
hold. I encourage my clients to use alternative methods to
curl and style the hair, too, without having to use heat.
Use soft scrunchies on freshly dried hair rolled around
your finger and secured in sections with each scrunchy.
Heat gently with a hair dryer, let go cold and then shake
the hair out. This gives great modern movement to your
style without having to use curling tongs.*

*'A great blow dry by your hairdresser can also have lon-
gevity and look great all week.'*

Colouring Hair

*'Ask your stylist to design a low-maintenance colour.
Hairdressers are generally taught to colour all over; this
often is not necessary and you can get great results without touching your scalp. So challenge your hairdresser to
think out of the box. You are in charge, you are paying
the expert.'*

If you aren't lucky enough to be near a salon offering organic
and mineral colours, then there are a few things you can do
to minimize your exposure to potentially toxic chemicals.

For starters, leave as long as you can between colouring
sessions and opt for high- or lowlights rather than full-head
colouring. If you want to colour your own hair at home
there are some good natural hair colours, but you will still
need to accept that these aren't 100 per cent natural. You
may also find that while the plant-based dyes can provide
excellent vibrant colours, which cover grey well, they can

sometimes give a kind of 'staining effect' and aren't always as conditioning as conventional brands. They can also give a rather matt appearance rather than the shiny look you may be used to. Try some brands out:

- www.logona.co.uk
- www.herbatint.co.uk
- www.naturesdream.co.uk

Nature's Dream permanent hair colour doesn't contain ammonia, resorcinol or parabens and their temporary colour rinse is also free from peroxide and PPDs. Girlfriends have told me it's great for grey hair. They offer an excellent free phone consultation service, too, 0845 6018129.

Natural Shampoo and Conditioner

There are some great natural shampoos and conditioners out there. Try:

- www.essential-care.co.uk
- www.greenpeople.co.uk
- www.soorganic.com

And check out the Shikakai natural shampoo powder www.rawgaia.com.

Girlfriends' Natural Secrets ... I make a scrub for an itchy scalp. Pop a few tablespoons of brown sugar, the same of olive oil and 5 drops each of tea tree, rosemary and lavender essential oils in a bowl and mix up. When I'm in the bath I work that all through my scalp to loosen dry skin; the olive oil then gets to work to moisturize. By the time I've read a bit and finished the glass of wine, it has done the job. I wash this out by applying the shampoo straight onto my hair before I get it near water, that way the oil can be properly washed out. I don't need conditioner after this, it's just silky soft hair and itch-free.

– Emily www.purenuffstuff.co.uk

DIY HAIRCARE

Luscious shiny hair comes from within but in addition to eating the right foods you can often apply them to your hair and get great results!

Here are some ideas for shampoos, conditioners, rinses and treatments, but let's start with hair oil. I have only recently started using the amazing hair oil from John Masters Organics and it has given me the confidence to start to blend my own for use on my hair and scalp. For itchy hair try:

Dandruff Treatment Oil
– 50 ml almond oil
– 5 drops rosemary essential oil
– 5 drops lavender oil
– 5 drops cedarwood oil

Apply to the scalp, leave on for an hour before washing off with a natural shampoo. Then rinse with one of the rinses listed on page 61.

Girlfriends Natural Secrets … Make a conditioning hair oil: mix 20 drops of rosemary, 20 drops of geranium and 10 of lavender oil in 100 ml of olive oil. Massage it into your scalp. Leave it in all day if you can (I just tie back my hair and enjoy the aroma all day!). Wash off and feel the silkiness!

– Ayse Georgiou

DIY Shampoo

Shampoo can be tricky simply because of the high water content/preservative issue. It's best, therefore, simply to make enough for only one application. A simple idea is to use Castile liquid soap as a shampoo base and add herbal infusions and essential oils, or you could use soapnut liquid (more on this later).

If you do make more and need to store it, then remember the golden rule: if it's got water in it, then you'll need a preservative if it's going to be stored. You can use 2 drops of grapefruit seed extract liquid which you can find in health shops.

Here are a couple of simple ideas for homemade shampoos. Bear in mind, though, that homespun shampoos, especially those made with egg, won't foam up or create that lovely lather that we're all used to in our commercial shampoos. Don't worry about that; the solution will still clean the hair! Many of the more natural shampoos sold in health shops or online often don't foam up either, simply because they don't contain the harsh detergent foaming agents, so it's a good reason to get used to non-foaming washes generally.

Eggy Shampoo

This is great for dry hair and so quick to make.

- 1 egg yolk
- 100 ml herbal infusion

Whisk the egg yolk into the herbal infusion such as chamomile (I use a couple of chamomile tea bags). Massage it through your hair, leave for a couple of minutes and then rinse through with lukewarm water.

If you have oily hair, replace the egg yolk with egg white and follow the same instructions.

Soapnut Shampoo

Soapnut liquid makes a fantastic shampoo (see page 246 for more information on soapnuts).

Put 2 handfuls of soapnuts into a saucepan and add enough water to make it 1 part soapnuts to 3 parts water. Bring to the boil and then simmer for about 15 minutes.

When the soapnuts are really soft, strain off the liquid, allow it to cool and add a couple of drops of essential oil. This really is essential as the soapnut liquid doesn't smell that fantastic (my poor husband looked most forlorn when he came in, smelled the soapnuts simmering and thought this was going to be his dinner!). You can then whisk the solution up using a hand blender and – voilà – a fantastic shampoo (and indeed, a natural detergent that can be used for cleaning any surface or even the car!).

This will store well, so you can increase the quantities and store in a container with a lid.

Hair Conditioner

The best deep-conditioning hair treatment is, of course, organic coconut oil. You can apply it before you wash as a pre-conditioner which will leave hair very silky, or use it as a deep treatment after washing and leave on overnight, wrapping your hair in a towel or a protective bathcap. You'll need a couple of washes to remove it but it's well worth it. If you're going to be out in the sun it's very protective, too. You can coat your hair in coconut oil, tie it back, and when you wash it out you'll have lovely, silky hair that isn't sun-damaged.

Lots of the face mask ideas in the last chapter can be used as hair conditioners as well. Adding an egg yolk makes them very creamy. Here's a simple one that gets great results.

Avocado Hair Conditioner
    ½ avocado
- 1 teaspoon jojoba oil
- yolk of 1 egg

Mash the avocado with the jojoba oil. Add the egg yolk and blend in a high-speed blender. Apply and leave on for a few minutes, then rinse off.

Hair Rinse
- 1 chamomile tea bag
- 1 pint water

Steep the tea bag in the water for a great rinse especially for blonde hair.

For an Itchy Scalp
- 20 ml apple cider vinegar
- 100 ml water
- 3 drops rosemary oil
- 3 drops lavender oil

This is great for making the hair shiny and helping with an itchy, irritated scalp. You can also get fresh rosemary, steep it in hot water, allow to cool and then use as a rinse – excellent for dandruff and psoriasis.

The juice of half a lemon in water is good for fair hair, especially if it's oily. If you have dark hair, beer works well as a final rinse (better to use it up that way than to drink it!).

Between Shampoos

You already know I advocate leaving your hair as long as possible between washes. If you feel you just need to refresh the scalp area, you can use cotton wool and just a tiny amount of pure witch hazel and lavender water, wiping gently down your scalp.

If it's a spritz of good old dry shampoo you're after (if I'm ever having my hair styled for TV or for photos, make-up artists usually apply this first as it makes it easier to get flyaway hair to stay in place) then ditch the chemical version and make your own.

DIY Dry Shampoo
- 2 tablespoons arrowroot powder (you can buy this in health shops)
- 2 tablespoons cornstarch
- 10 drops of lavender or tea tree oil

Mix together, apply to your scalp, massage in quickly and then brush out thoroughly.

Hair Spray

Even if you aren't usually sensitive to synthetic chemicals, you're sure to have been overwhelmed at some point by the onslaught of regular hairsprays and their heady mix of potentially toxic fixative pongs. Try making your own:

DIY Hairspray
- 25 ml filtered water
- 25 ml lemon juice
- 10 g of sugar
- 1 drop vodka

Add to a small pump spray bottle and spritz away! If it doesn't seem to 'fix', add more sugar.

HAIR REMOVAL

There's no easy way round this one – well, at least, none that doesn't hurt. I'm lucky enough to be very fair so my hairy bits don't look so bad (in truth my eyesight isn't great either, so I could be deluding myself!). If it's an issue for you, though, I'd highly recommend *threading*, especially for facial hair.

Threading

This technique was developed in the Middle East and uses pure cotton held between the fingers and around rows of hair – sounds terrifying, doesn't it?, but I know several girl-friends who have found skilful practitioners who are adept at threading for removing facial hair, and especially for eye-brow shaping. It's quicker, less painful than many other techniques, and chemical-free, so ask around for a recommendation in case there's a salon offering it near you.

Waxing

Waxing is probably the most obvious form of hair removal, but opt for a salon using natural waxes rather than petro-chemical-based ones if possible. There are also many organic alternatives now on the market from companies like:

- www.soorganic.com
- www.moom-uk.com

Sugaring

Sugaring is making a comeback, too. It's been used in the Middle East for ever and a day. You can make your own sugaring solution with lemon juice, sugar and glycerine. I have to admit that just the thought of heating this mixture up, applying it (you use fabric strips) and then stripping it off makes me shudder! I prefer to spend money and put myself in the hands of a trained therapist, preferably one who doesn't mind hearing me squeal!

Just a word about regular depilatory creams for home hair removal: I'd avoid if possible, most contain some harsh chemicals. Why do you think they smell so bad?

TEETH

Toothpaste

The whole fluoride debate is too lengthy to get into here (see my articles on www.imperfectlynatural.com), but whether or not you decide to opt for fluoride, you'd be well advised to avoid the foaming agents and other nasties in regular toothpastes.

There are lots of natural ones depending on your favourite tastes. Try Green People, Kingfisher, Sarakan, Tom's of Maine – all available in health shops. The only ones that aren't in health shops are perhaps the most natural of all: the lemon or mint flavours from Miessence (www.mionegroup.com) and the Kiki Aloe Ferox tooth gel (www.fresh-network.com). For toothpastes free from fluoride, aluminium, artificial sweeteners or detergents, try www.sheerorganics.com or www.janeysnaturalstore.co.uk.

Avoid conventional toothpaste where you can and opt to

make your own. Bicarbonate of soda, water and salt are the main ingredients, but you can experiment to taste.

Toothpaste
- 1 tablespoon bicarbonate of soda
- pinch Himalayan salt
- 1 teaspoon lemon juice
- 1 drop peppermint essential oil

Add enough filtered water to mix the ingredients to form a paste. This will harden if left, so keep in an airtight container and use within a day or so.

You can also buy a 'natural toothbrush' – basically a twig that contains minerals – looks ridiculous but perfect for when you're travelling: www.organ-nics.com.

HANDS AND NAILS
I'm afraid I'm imperfect here, gals. My nails are tatty and, somehow, however healthy my diet is, they seem to break and split. They also, for some inexplicable reason, always seem to be dirty and give the appearance that I've just been gardening – it's not a good look but I'm laying my cards on the table. Confessions notwithstanding, of course I must tell you that your nails are a mirror of what's going on within, but also need regular tender loving care. Gloves are one answer, of course. Personally I hate wearing them for cleaning (you just can't feel the corners), but I'm becoming used to the necessity, and for nails I believe that, rather like facial oils, nail oils are the way forward. If you shape and buff your nails regularly and use a tiny drop of nail oil, that will help them tremendously.

It won't surprise you to know that most nail polishes are a fairly scary mix of toxic chemicals. You'll recognize the whiff, I'm sure, as they usually contain toluene, formaldehyde and solvents, alcohol and much more. Fortunately you can get great ranges of water-based polishes which don't contain the very harsh chemicals.

Suncoat and Sante are the market leaders; their water-based nail polishes are coloured naturally with earth pigments (vegan where possible) rather than synthetic dyes.

Application

Beware, though, as the technique for applying these natural varnishes is different from what you're used to. You don't need a base coat and you often need three coats, as they create a (non-staining!) film over the nail. And remember they're water-based, so you need first to have removed any traces of oil.

Be aware, too, that your regular nail varnish remover won't remove water-based polishes. In fact, if I'm truthful I find natural nail polishes a devil to get off – the easiest way is to pick it off! Charming, I know! But you can also use a special remover such as one from Suncoat made from a mixture of soy and maize ingredients. It's completely natural, vegan and biodegradable and it *contains no acetone or acetates*. The good news is that you can use it to remove conventional polish too; its oily consistency won't dry nails out.

- Suncoat www.allergybestbuys.co.uk
- Sante www.spiritofnature.co.uk
- Elysambre www.kinetic4health.co.uk
- Nubar www.cultbeauty.co.uk

If you're lucky enough to live near Herefordshire, Oxfordshire or Hertfordshire, you can get a natural expert manicure courtesy of salons such as:

- Spirit Organic www.spiritorganic.com
- Pure Me in Farringdon
- Green Hands in Leominster www.greenhands.co.uk
- Jenny's Nails mobile nail technician in Herts www.jennysnails.info

Our hands show our age, of course. Treat yourself to regular hand massages. You can do your own using 100 per cent natural creams. See the info on coconut oil (page 10), slather it on and wear gloves overnight. The next day your hands will be soft and silky.

Hand and Nail Care

It's simple to make your own hand cream or oil using any of the recipes already suggested for facial oils or creams. Of course a rich barrier cream will require lanolin, beeswax or even glycerine, but if you want to keep it really simple it's back to the good old coconut oil! You can add essential oils to give it some fragrance.

Pampering Hand Oil
- 10 ml avocado oil
- 10 drops carrot oil
- 10 drops jojoba oil
- 1 vitamin E capsule

Blend the oils together then add a few drops of your favourite essential oils. You could use 2 drops of lemon, 2 drops of lavender and 5 drops of rose, or try geranium. It's not an exact science – enjoy blending! Massage a tiny amount into your hands and they'll feel really soft.

Nails

Essential oils will stimulate nail growth and help to strengthen them.

Strengthening Blend
- 2 teaspoons avocado oil
- 5 drops jojoba oil
- 5 drops lemon oil
- 5 drops rosemary

Massage into fingernails or toenails.

To Enhance Nail Growth
- 100 ml sweet almond oil
- 20 drops lemon or grapefruit essential oil

Massage into nails to get the circulation going.

The Power of Fragrance

The sense of smell is incredibly important. Our fifth sense is apparently a thousand times more powerful than our sense of taste. Smells bring back memories, keep us healthy, lead to seduction and have a direct effect on the most primitive part of our brain, which is called the limbic system. The limbic brain is the seat of our emotions. Our feelings of fear and anxiety, happiness and contentment are all created in this part of the brain, and it controls emotions and memory. It is also connected to the endocrine and autonomic nervous systems, and it controls all functions of survival, including digestion, respiration, circulation and reproduction.

Every whiff that reaches our nose has an effect on our body, whether good or bad. Odours influence what we remember, how we feel, how we learn, whom we have sex with, even how often! Good aromas are therapeutic. I had my first aromatherapy massage and literally thought I'd died and gone to heaven. It wasn't merely 'pampering', though; much as I felt massaged and had a good sense of well-being I believe it was also healing. My aromatherapist used her intuition, and of course my symptoms, to determine which oils she needed to blend to keep me well. There were many occasions when I'd go in feeling very stressed and anxious, with aches and pains or flu-like symptoms, and emerge feeling confident and bursting with energy, with no sign of a cold!

AROMAS

Traditionally perfumes are made from plant and animal substances and prepared in the form of waters, oils, powders and incense. There is a huge difference between natural and synthetic fragrance, not only in what they are made from but, more critically, how they affect the body. Most modern perfumes are alcohol-based and contain 20 per cent or more synthetic scents. They are created by mixing a solvent, a fixative and a fragrant compound. The alcohol used is often of poor quality and can affect the liver and cause sensitizing skin reactions such as white spots when exposed to the sun.

I asked Petre Sefton, the founder of Tortue Rouge who runs perfume-making courses in rural France, to explain the differences between natural and synthetic fragrances and their effect on us. I attended one of these courses, and it was a wonderfully fun and inspiring experience.

'For centuries natural perfumes were created with scented oils extracted by pressing, pulverizing or distilling aromatic vegetable and animal substances. The fragrance of aromatic plants and trees originates as droplets of highly volatile non-greasy oil produced and stored in tiny glands located throughout the plant – in the rind of a fruit, the roots, resin or heartwood of a tree. These essential oils are powerful and effective tools to affect the mind and the emotions. Because they are made up of light, volatile chemicals they are easily and rapidly absorbed by the nasal mucosa with great therapeutic potential – physical and mental. Essential oils are expensive to produce, and it's no surprise that modern commerce sought cheaper chemical substitutes. They also often use solvents instead of distillation to extract precious scents.

Lift Your Spirits with Oils

'Therapists and psychologists are increasingly using essential oils in treatments. It is possible to completely alter your frame of mind in a matter of minutes with these precious essences of nature. Essential oils have an impact on both right and left hemispheres of the brain: the left brain, being the orderly, thinking brain, most alert during the day; the right brain, the creative side that deals with emotion and imagination, is more active at night. Natural fragrances can be engineered to affect one side of the brain more than the other, or even to act as a bridge between them. Natural fragrances also act on the pheromones, the natural chemical scents the body produces in order to communicate with others nearby. Their 'perfume' helps us tell lovers (actual and potential) and family members from strangers, and allows mothers and infants to bond.

'The natural fragrance molecules don't last as long as the synthetics because they are much more volatile. But they don't smother our own personal body fragrance, rather *they combine to make a unique glowing bouquet that speaks to our inner being via the limbic brain. Natural perfumery can be used for emotional communication and healing in a way that synthetic perfumery cannot.*

'Whilst the role of traditional perfumery is essentially aesthetic – to adorn and to attract – natural or 'spiritual' perfumery involves the adornment of the soul as well as of the body – with a goal not only to evoke beauty, but also to invoke inner harmony. A natural perfume, therefore, is a potential tool for emotional healing – as long as it is created with a sensitive understanding of the person who will wear it.'

MAKING AN 'AURIC' FRAGRANCE

You can make a natural fragrance by combining as few as three essential oils in a base of good quality sweet almond oil. This can then be used as a lotion to massage the body, too.

First you need the initial impact for a fragrance, known as the 'top note' or 'head note'. It's usually a light fragrance that gets your attention but then seems to die down after a few minutes. The middle or 'heart note' is deeper and more subtle and remains more constant in the fragrance. Then there's the 'base note', which underpins the other two and becomes more noticeable as the aroma of the other two starts to fade away. As you experiment, remember that smelling a perfume straight from the bottle is not the same as smelling it on your skin!

Recipes

Choose a head note, a heart note and a base note.

To give you an idea of which essential oils correspond with these notes, here's a rough guide.

- **Head notes** – lemon, oregano, orange, basil, bergamot, lavender, ylang ylang
- **Heart notes** – rose, geranium, cedarwood, chamomile, neroli, rosemary
- **Base notes** – clove, nutmeg, sandalwood, rosewood, clary sage, cinnamon, patchouli, ginger, juniper, black pepper

Find a few of each type of oil and lay them out in front of you. Smell them quickly and see if you can imagine how they might blend with the others, then experiment, making sure you have a small glass bottle to hand and essential oils with dropper bottles.

- Put 1 drop of each of the oils you choose, so one head, one heart, one base, into a tablespoon of sweet almond oil. Swirl it around and see if it's pleasing; if so, you can use a tiny bit dabbed on your wrist or in a massage oil.

Two Great Blends
- 2 drops grapefruit
- 2 drops rosemary
- 2 drops juniper
- 1 tablespoon sweet almond oil

This will be energizing and great to wear in the morning.

- 3 drops orange
- 3 drops neroli

- 1 drop sandalwood
- 1 tablespoon sweet almond oil

Wear this as a body 'lotion' and be seriously seductive!
Finally, a last word from Petre.

> *'Perfume is our visiting card, the fragrance we leave behind us. We choose our fragrance to reflect who we want to be or seem to be. Your perfume may not be saying what you wish, it might also be affecting your health. Please choose with care.'*

ESSENTIAL OILS AS REMEDIES

Of course essential oils can be incredibly therapeutic, not just as perfumes or lotions but as natural remedies for many ills.

- For a nose bleed: 1 drop *Cistus landiferus* on cotton wool applied to the nostrils will help stop the bleeding.
- To relieve travel sickness or insomnia during flying: 1 drop lavender oil on each wrist.
- To prevent that awful feeling of heavy and restless legs: 10 drops lemon essential oil and 10 drops of cyprus essential oil in 1 ounce hazelnut oil. Use this to massage your calves and thighs. You can do this for a day or so before a long-haul flight as well as during.
- For flu protection: ditch the hand sanitizers and make a simple, effective antiviral mix that can be used to spritz the air, as a hand wash or on the body. You need a couple of unusual oils for this but a good aromatherapy supplier should have them.
  - 10 ml essential oil of ravensara
  - 5 ml eucalyptus radiata (it's specifically antiviral)

At the first sign of flu or cold symptoms, rub 15 drops of this neat essential oil mix on the throat and 15 drops on the lower back three times a day for around 3 days. Dilute the mix in some distilled water to make a sprizter to spray around your personal space. (I like using this on aircraft especially to refresh the air) and you can put 10 to 20 drops in an ounce of aloe vera gel to make an antiviral hand rub.

To source good quality oils:

- www.tortuerouge.com
- www.justaromatherapy.co.uk
- www.eoco.org.uk
- www.potions.co.uk
- www.beautyasbliss.com

See the section on DIY recipes (starting on page 33) for more uses for essential oils in skincare. For soapmaking and perfumery courses see www.organic-courses.com.

Please bear in mind that if you suffer allergies or are pregnant or breastfeeding, you should consult a health practitioner before you use essential oils.

Girlfriends' Natural Secrets . . . My absolute favourite natural skincare ingredient is natural yoghurt – just as it is, it's a fabulous cleanser. Add some sugar for an exfoliating skin rub (or oats for a gentler, conditioning rub), or use it as a facepack with honey (all types), mashed avocado (dry skin) or chopped fresh tomatoes (oily skin).

– Helen Prudames www.purenuffstuff.co.uk

Janey's Guide to Exercise

MOVE YOUR BODY!

I reserve the right to change my mind. It's a woman's prerogative, so they say, and exercise is one area where I've completely changed my attitude over the last few years. I now realize that even moderate regular exercise will slow down the ageing process and boost energy levels. I've never been a sporty type, though. I'm unsure whether I just don't have the frame for running and sprinting, but I also lack the competitive spirit and genuinely have never had any interest in team games or keeping fit, probably not helped by humiliation in school PE lessons. For years the closest I got to exercise was moving my fingers to dial phone numbers – well, I did do some ballet, but I certainly did not partake in aerobic exercise of any kind. So what changed my mind? Well, finally realizing that exercise has so many physical and mental benefits. Several studies have found that a lifestyle that includes regular exercise could prevent 14 per cent of male and 20 per cent of female cancer deaths in the UK alone.

As Christopher Reeve said on television, addressing particularly the growing number of obese viewers:

> *'The one thing that you all can do is movement. Those of you that have the gift of movement that don't use it, is an insult to those of us who have lost that ability, it's the one thing I'd love to do more than anything on earth, I'd gladly be 500 lb overweight; give me three years and I'd lose it because I'd move my body every day.'*

I now move *my* body every day because I'm able to, and as you age you eventually realize that you're able to only *because* you've moved your body every day! You wouldn't really expect an old car to start if you left it stationary for years; similarly, *your* starter motor needs regular revving up – and no, moving three paces to grab the remote control won't cut it.

FINDING SOMETHING YOU ENJOY

It's really a mindset change and it's about finding something you enjoy. By moving my body I don't necessarily mean working out in the gym. That suits some people and good on you if you enjoy that. Personally I find running on a treadmill and using those rowing machines very unnatural and, in truth, I think many gyms are rather unhealthy. If that sounds like a bizarre statement, think of the sweaty aerobics studios which often have those automatic air 'freshening' devices fitted. They release a potentially toxic artificial fragrance into a room full of people breathing deeply (at the gym I tried we were practising full yogic breathing when it kicked in). And have you ever tried to grab a snack at the gym café? Most stock a whole range of calorie-laden sugary snacks and, worse still, often have big marketing campaigns for diet and so called 'isotonic' sports drinks which contain artificial sweeteners (you'll hear more about my very strong views on that subject later on!) and artificial flavours and colours.

I'm not including, by the way, in my aversion to gyms, those 'ladies' gyms' which have opened up now such as Curves. They offer a carefully designed circuit of weight-bearing machines which take just 30 minutes to complete and are said to offer both toning and aerobic fitness in one go. That worked for me for a few months and, being local to me at the time, there was no faffing about having to get adorned in fancy gym kit and then showering in the changing rooms and almost keeling over at the chemical soup of fragrances people were spraying around.

NO TIME?

Lack of time is the reason most of us give for not exercising, but that's really no excuse, we all have the same number of hours, it's just how we utilize them. After my first juice detox retreat I was introduced to the rather new concept of enjoying two 6 o'clocks in one day! I started getting up much earlier and exercising while the rest of the family slumbered. You can also, of course, use exercise in place of public transport. Cycling is the obvious one but that's not for the faint-hearted if you're an urban city-dwelling girlfriend.

WALKING IS THE NEW RUNNING

For the very-quick-to-get-out-of-breath-and-feel-miserable runners like me, you'll be pleased to know you can get just as effective a workout from very brisk walking, with the added benefit of arriving at your destination relatively unsweaty, thus saving on travel costs and time needed for showering. You're probably aware that 10,000 steps a day is the recommended you need to achieve, so it's clear that that quarter-of-a-mile stroll to the wine bar won't cut it. If you aim to walk for at least 30 minutes at a brisk pace, and you swing your arms into the bargain (leave the designer handbag at home and invest in a light backpack if you must carry stuff; Jimmy Choos aren't recommended either, get yourself some comfortable trainers), you'll notice a difference in how toned you feel in a very short space of time.

Personal trainer Estella Ramos says:

'Keeping your body moving is fundamental for your health and well-being even if it is just walking, as the benefits are second to none. Use the outdoors to get muscles working. The woods are a great place for this, as uneven ground is great for working those calf muscles and getting the heart rate up! If I am just out walking locally I like to pick up the pace, holding my stomach muscles in with a good posture. As my mum would say, "Chin up, shoulders back, best foot forward!" In fact, up until recently my mum never walked anywhere and drove everywhere, until she had quite a nasty car accident and now she doesn't drive but walks everywhere. Struggling on a daily basis with arthritis, the pace to start with was slow. She walks to her local supermarket, which used to take her 45 minutes. By picking up the pace gradually she now makes it in 15 minutes. In seven months she has lost 2½ stone and is more energized, experiences less pain and is happier and slimmer!

'By picking up the pace of your walk, your heart rate rises and your lungs work harder, which will reduce the chance of getting any cardiovascular diseases. You burn

*more fat, feel more energized and get to where you want
to go in half the time!'*

I recently tried a Nordic walking session at a spa. 'How hard
can it be?' I thought, 'I can walk, can't I? How can holding
a couple of long walking "rods" cramp my style?' Well perhaps I shouldn't have been so cocky. Nordic walking is really
quite tricky til you get the knack, but what it does reveal
is your posture and how co-ordinated you are at swinging
alternate arms to legs, if you get my drift. There are Nordic
walking clubs all over now, and Champneys offer regular
walking retreats to help you to find ways to improve your
fitness levels just by putting one foot in front of the other.

I'm guessing there won't be a girlfriend who hasn't heard
of special MBT trainers or Fitflops. The principle is that they
help to tone up the muscles as you walk. MBT trainers (Masai
Barefoot Technology; www.uk.mbt.com) force the sole of the
foot into a kind of rolling action; in fact when I first wore
mine I felt slightly seasick as I rocked back and forth, but
you soon get used to the sensation. It's worth persevering if
they feel weird, as they're said to improve muscle function and
make any workout almost 40 per cent more effective! They're
not cheap, at around £150, but if you shop around you might
find a bargain on eBay or in a charity shop like I did!

Girlfriends' Aspirations . . . To run a 10k road
race next year. I've just taken up running again after two
bouts of breast cancer and am determined to get fit again.
Also to keep focused on the important things in life and not
get hung up on the latest handbag or new top. Make time to
smell the roses and be with the people that matter.

I read this quote today: 'Life isn't about waiting for the storm to pass. It's about learning to dance in the rain!' ... Really like that!

– Susan J Thomson

OTHER WAYS OF KEEPING FIT

If you want to do more than running or walking there are literally hundreds of different fitness activities at your disposal now. Depending on where you live, you could find yourself round the corner from a wealth of possibilities as diverse as funky ballet, fitball, salsa and hula-hooping through tennis and kick-boxing. Then of course there are lots of ways you can keep fit with only a tiny outlay cost-wise at home.

Rebounding

I highly recommend rebounding. If you haven't heard about this joyous way of keeping fit before now, listen up. My rebounder for many years was merely another receptacle to drape clothes over, until I experienced the delight of my first rebounding class on a detox retreat. Jason Vale, the juice guru who was running the retreat, leaps at least 4 feet into the air (don't try this at home unless your ceilings are high!) and his enthusiasm is infectious. He looks rather like a smile on the end of an elastic band, but this is one activity that you don't have to be especially good at, nor especially fit, nor do you need any skill or technique, you simply bounce, up and down, side to side, using your arms. You can be young or old, or even have minor injuries.

Rebounding helps with detoxification, and will not only tone you up but afford you better energy levels and clearer skin. It's the best all-around aerobic exercise that one can do vertically – i.e. second only to swimming. All the organs are stimulated, and it's fantastic for lymphatic drainage but with the huge advantage that there's no getting wet involved and no chlorine to play havoc with your hair. It's also popular with NASA, who have stated that 'Rebounding is the most efficient and effective exercise yet devised by man.'

Doing a rebounding class overlooking the mountains in southern Turkey listening to Jason Vale's cheesy choice of music tracks took some beating, but I persevered and now use my rebounder daily. Sometimes while the kids bounce on their proper trampoline I bounce on mine (of course I can't go on theirs – I've got my pelvic floor to think about, for god's sake!). The trick is put on some music that you love or even watch TV while you bounce; 15 minutes' worth of bouncing is one heck of a good workout and, trust me, it's impossible not to smile and feel a sense of elation while bouncing – remember Tigger from Winnie the Pooh?

You can buy a rebounder from as little as £25 in high street or department stores, but for a great quality one go to www.juicemaster.com. They sell the Probounce or the more expensive but really amazing Bellicon.

Hula Hoops

The aforementioned hula hoop is a cheap, easy bit of exercise kit you can have at home. The best ones are slightly weighted and there's all kinds of intricate moves you can do to keep the hoop spinning!

> The right exercise for you changes your state
> of mind. For you it might be rowing, cycling,
> swimming – it doesn't matter. The best exercise for
> you is the one you feel like doing every day.

Girlfriends' Natural Secrets . . . *My beauty
secret is dance; I love to dance! I could dance for hours. For
me dancing is a form of expression that comes from within.
It is one of the only forms of exercise that gets my body
moving for hours without noticing. I sweat, I work every
muscle in my body, I grow in confidence, I burn a shed-load
of calories and it makes me smile, which I feel is the key to
looking and feeling youthful.*

— **Estella Ramos, personal trainer**

YOGA

Yoga is so very much more than simply exercise. Since attending regular classes I've improved my muscle tone, balance, breathing, posture and stamina. Yoga has so many
benefits including reducing stress levels, boosting the immune system, helping with body coordination, encouraging
mindfulness (more of this later), improving self-confidence
and self-discipline, and so much more. People who practise yoga regularly often find it easier to maintain their ideal
weight, and it helps with skin tone.

You don't have to be 'good' at yoga; you can work entirely
to your own ability, and over the couple of years I've been
practising, even though I have 'improved', with yoga there's
no specific goal or standard to adhere to. There are experts

who can wrap their legs around their neck and do all kinds of supple movements – I doubt if I'll ever manage that – but whatever you do in yoga will be beneficial. When I practise yoga it's not in order to win any prizes, it's only for my own benefit and I only really notice how 'rusty' I've become when I stop practising for a while.

I used to find yoga too repetitive, but there are many different types of yoga and even within the disciplines each teachers teaches differently. Try and find a good yoga teacher whom you feel an affinity with. I was lucky enough to find the amazing Matt Gluck (yoga mat!) who offers a wide range of different yoga techniques in his classes so it's never boring. He also adds a subtle spiritual element, too: most classes end with breathing postures and a guided meditative relaxation.

Here is Matt's wonderfully enthusiastic account of why yoga is so special for him:

> *'Yoga is harmony. When yoga finds you, it is because your heart has sent an internal call for help. It comes in the form of teachers who love sharing the truth of their own journey. During this voyage you see your real self. It's so familiar and you laugh and cry because you know you've always been here waiting.*

> *'Yoga releases your life, so that you shine again from the inside. You start to let go of useless emotions and destructive thoughts. They are replaced by bubbling JOY that wells from within the core of your being as you remember that you are here for a reason. You dance around again like a five-year-old child, gleaming with excitement to*

share your message. This happiness and contentment of heart lead to true vitality.

'Health emanates from within your cells, as they laugh in symphony, playing for a united whole once again.'

– Matt Gluck www.pranasanayoga.co.uk

A great place to start with yoga is to understand the emphasis the practice puts on *breathing*. Here's Matt again:

'A wonderful key to the breath is to LET GO with the exhalation – allow your body–mind to feel heavy, as though it is moving downwards, with the gravitational pull of the earth.

*'**Exhale** with the feeling of letting go at the end of a busy day, or putting down a load of heavy shopping.*

*'**Inhale** allowing your body–mind to feel light, as though it is lifting upwards away from the earth.*

'When you are heavy and grounded, you feel stable and calm. When you feel light and buoyant, you feel free and uplifted. Both exercises prove to us that our breathing has a direct relationship with our outlook, and that our outlook affects our breathing.

'Whether we are inhaling or exhaling, we are looking to be relaxed, as this facilitates even circulation and distribution of blood and oxygen within the joints, connective tissues, organs and glands. As you progress and combine these exercises with limbering practices, relaxation and vitality are sure to come.'

Ideally it's good to do your own short yoga practice at home a few times a week. I must confess I sometimes find that hard; there always seem to be distractions. Recently, though, I've learned about the series of moves called the Five Tibetans Rite of Rejuvenation. It consists of five exercises, each of which is performed 21 times (but this can be built up to over time). The whole practice takes about 12 minutes, so fits any schedule!

Yoga Guru Ken Ryan explains the technique:

Begin with a short gentle warm-up, rolling your shoulders and neck, stretching out your hamstrings, rolling forward, etc.

1. Spinning – with arms at shoulder level, spin 21 times in a clockwise direction. Remember doing this as a child?! You will feel a bit giddy, but don't go so fast that you fall over! When you finish, stand still and breathe gently.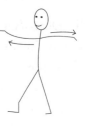

2. Leg raises – Supporting your pelvis with your hands joined at the tailbone, lift your legs from the horizontal to the vertical plane. Bend forward so your forehead moves towards your knees, inhale to bend, exhale to release. Practise with bent knees if you have any weakness in your lower back.

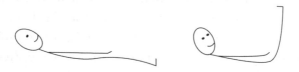

3. Camel – Kneeling upright with hands behind hips, press the pelvis forward, lifting the sternum. Look up, then return to the upright position. Inhale to lift, exhale back to the vertical position.

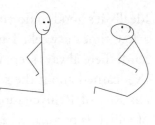

4. Table – From a sitting position with legs stretched long, and hands by your hips, lift up by bending your knees and raising your torso.

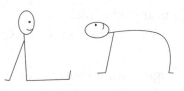

Lift until your body is vertical from knees to shoulders, looking up. Inhale to rise, exhale to lower and sit again.

5. Down/Up Dog – Begin in Downward Dog position: hands and feet forming a

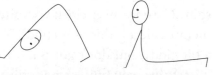

long base on the ground, pelvis lifted as high as possible, legs, back and arms straight. Move into Upward Dog by shifting your weight forward towards your hands, releasing your pelvis down while energetically arching your spine to lift your chest. Inhale as you move forward, exhale back to Downward Dog.

****

Any yoga practice you do regularly will benefit you, so try to familiarize yourself with a few postures and do them daily. If you work at a desk most of the day, take a few minutes out, preferably once every few hours, and do a few stretches – Downward Dog is excellent, and should give your colleagues across the office a laugh!

- For great diagrams of yoga positions see the marvellous book *The Yoga Bible: Definitive Guide to Yoga Postures* by Christina Brown
- Great yoga DVDs include *Journey to Tranquillity* by Ken Ryan – available from www.juicemaster.com

Girlfriends' Natural Secrets . . . *I try to fit in a 5-minute routine every day, doing all the things you hear you should do once a day but never actually do unless you make time. Examples of the things I do include: a 55-second spine stretch upon waking, a minute's 'Plank' (yoga posture) to strengthen my core muscles.*

Girlfriends' Aspirations . . . *I'd like to compile my own 'bucket list' to include places to visit, subjects to learn, activities to try, etc. and tick off the list, one by one before I kick the bucket ...*

– Clairey Meadowcroft

DANCING

I'm thrilled it's hip again to dance – the popularity of dancing shows on TV has really changed dance to something for the masses. All it takes is for you to find an opportunity, whether that be in your front room to your favourite music or in a club. I LOVE the guilty pleasures nights www.guiltypleasures.co.uk – you can relive your youth dancing the night away to great pop music, and dress up to boot. Or indeed you could attend a contemporary dance class. Many gyms and community centres are now offering hula hoop classes – there's certainly some tricky choreography to follow whilst balancing your hoop – through to funky or fusion ballet, which is fantastic for toning up legs and bums, and yet such great fun you feel like a child again.

The trick if you try any dance class – unless, of course, you are Darcy Bussell – is to simply forget what you look like, ignore studio mirrors (other than to check your posture) and simply enjoy the feeling of movement. Don't get into comparisons – Oh, and NEVER under any circumstances invite partners to critique your performance. My girlfriend's less than sensitive boyfriend came to meet her after her ballet fusion class and said she'd looked like one of the elephants from *Fantasia*! It may not surprise you to know she ditched the class (though I reckon she should have ditched the boyfriend!).

Girlfriends' Aspirations . . . To work on the shape of my legs, so my knees look like knees and not puddings! I am on the chunky side but have been losing weight and am very healthy. I have always been pretty active but my knees prevent me from wearing anything like shorts. I don't think I would go back to wearing a mini-skirt like in my early twenties ... but it would be nice to wear shorts on holiday or at the gym without feeling conscious about my knees.

– Lynne Gale, 51, businesswoman and aspiring author

NIA

I've recently found the most wonderful class. It's not really dance, it's more like movement with a bit of tai chi, yoga and eurythmy thrown into the mix.

Nia is a Swahili word meaning 'with purpose' and it's all about joyous movement to become healthy. It's also short for *Neuromuscular Integrative Action*, all done barefoot, and its grounded approach is said to maximize body efficiency and teach you to move consciously in a gentler way. It's said to help you approach everything 'with purpose, feeling passion and electricity'.

The first time I attended a Nia class I think I was expecting it to be rather like the kind of 'movement to music' I had done in school as a child, floating around being a 'tree in the wind'. Nothing had prepared me for the wonderfully eclectic fusion of yoga, martial arts, modern and ethnic dance. It's all done to great music and you're encouraged to visualize and focus your energy in such a way that you really do need to be 'present'. There is structured choreography, it's definitely dance-based, but it allows for freedom of expression in movement and individual creativity, too. You don't have to be especially light on your feet or adept at following tricky movements.

It was created by Debbie and Carlos Rosa in 1983 after they were searching for a pleasurable way to keep fit that also frees the body from physical tensions while strengthening the heart and mind. They say it promotes strength and muscle definition without the use of weights, and its freeing, dance-like nature provides a medium for self-healing. You'll tighten, tone, lengthen, strengthen, lose pounds and inches – and have fun while you're doing it.

There are more than 100 Nia trainers in the UK (www.uknia.com), so seek one out and enjoy!

GETTING MOTIVATED

When starting any exercise programme, having something to aim for really helps get you motivated. Choose a realistic goal – perhaps a holiday or special party you're going to in a few months' time – and visualize yourself looking fantastic in the photographs. It's well documented that athletes who visualize themselves beating their personal best usually do, as opposed to those who simply train hard and hope they'll do well.

You may also want to offer yourself rewards for when you meet your goals – but don't make it a large chocolate bar. Opt for a sparkly mineral eyeshadow or natural nail polish instead. If you feel you need someone else to motivate you, find a personal trainer you feel in tune with. As always, ask around for someone local to you who shares the same ideals of health and well-being.

PASSIVE EXERCISE

Yes, there are some exercises you can do without actually doing anything.

The Chi Machine (www.thechimachine.co.uk) is basically a 'no impact, no effort' exerciser. You simply lie back, place your feet on the foot rests, plug it in and wobble away. It feels very weird at first because your whole body swivels, but you can build up your time over the first few weeks of use and it starts to feel very comfortable. Apparently 15 minutes of 'massage' on a chi machine is equivalent to 90 minutes' brisk walking because of the oxygenation of the blood, so it's suitable for the elderly, those with arthritic pain and those who can't do regular exercise, as well as girlfriends who simply want to lie back and relax while they get the benefit of improved circulation, less stress, relief from headaches, better posture, better sleep and balanced digestion. It can even aid weight loss and result in firmer and more toned thighs and buttocks (yep, that was the deciding factor for me!). Some hospitals in Japan rate the Chi Machine as an important clinical and medical health appliance.

VIBRATE YOURSELF FIT!

You'll also have heard, of course, about vibration platforms. There are various brands including the Vibrogym and the Power Plate often found now in gyms. It's the so-called 'celebrity workout' because it affords you a full workout in 15 minutes. It's not just a gimmick, either: they were originally used in Russia for cosmonauts heading off into space, and later to train athletes. Try and think of it as another aid to toning rather than a quick fix on its own, but undoubtedly it's a useful tool and quite fun if you like that 'vibrating' feeling. The local centre where my little girl does street dancing also has a Power Plate: I drop her off and have exactly 20 minutes to wobble away – that's better than nattering with the other mums in the café – well maybe not, but it's better for my butt and bingo wings. Check before you use vibration platforms, though, as they are not suitable for everyone, and if possible get a training session before you use one.

FIND A FRIEND!

I moved house recently and had no idea where I could go for long walks locally. I'm not good with Ordnance Survey maps so that wasn't an option for me, so I did a very unBritish thing: I set off on a walk, got to my local common and then asked another woman if she would mind pointing me in the direction of a decent easy route to walk. She went one better: she came with me! She's become my regular walking partner and we motivate each other. However late I go to bed I know she's setting her alarm to meet me for a brisk walk in all weathers so I can't let her down.

If you've got a dog, that's a great excuse to do two long walks every day.

See if there are local walking groups in your area, or just ask around your friends and neighbours. There are also lots of running networks – join one! If you've made a date to exercise you're far more likely to stick to your goals. Try www.womensrunningnetwork.co.uk.

RELAXING AFTER EXERCISE

I must admit I had never heard of acupressure mats or similar until I received the Shakti Mat to review. At first it looked a little scary: a plastic mat with lots of tiny plastic needles sticking out! I read the instructions with some trepidation as to quite what I was meant to do with it. The Shakti Mat is a modern take on the traditional Indian 'bed of nails', with roots going back to the 5,000-year-old Vedic tradition – the practice of attaining perfect balance of body, mind and spirit. The mat has 6,000 acupressure points which make it wonderful for releasing tension and inducing a state of deep relaxation. When you use the Shakti Mat regularly for 20 to 40 minutes, you enable your body to release endorphins which stimulate the release of oxytocin, the 'feel-good hormone'. As a result, your body relaxes and releases stress, promoting restful sleep and relieving stressful back and neck pain. The first few times I used it I needed to lay a thin cloth over the top – I was such a wimp – but after a while you do get used to the tingling sensation and it certainly does feel relaxing. www.shaktimat.co.uk

Janey's Guide to Ethical Fashion

I've already hinted that one of the most ethical fashionista 'styles' is to go retro and charity-shop chic. There's nothing more green than reusing what you or someone else has already worn for ages, and a whole new industry has grown up around revitalizing your clothing and reworking old garments into new. The wartime 'make do and mend' approach is back with a vengeance, and even if you aren't handy with a needle and thread there's no reason why you can't use pins (even safety pins – remember the punk era?), Velcro and various other ways of changing what you already have and adding accessories to create a whole new look. Even the iconic Vivienne Westwood is now recommending that we stop compulsive buying and rediscover creativity within our wardrobes. She suggests making our own outfits or adapting what we have by using old curtains and revamping with buttons and old jewellery.

BUYING NEW

If you like to buy new, consider the real cost of the almost disposable 'fast fashion' in some of the high street stores. Ask yourself where it was made and who was slaving over it for hours to earn a penny. And what's in the fabric? Many seemingly innocuous cotton T-shirts are from GM crops, lots of materials have been bleached and dyed using harsh synthetic dyes, or have suffered some kind of chemical treatment. Growing cotton takes more pesticides than any other single crop. This is nothing new, of course: the expression 'mad as a hatter' came about because people who made hats in the 19th century absorbed so many toxic chemicals and heavy metals that it affected their brains.

Ask yourself, too, whether you really need that new item of clothing. It's estimated that in the UK women spend over £5 billion on clothes that they will never wear. Nearly 75 per cent of the two million tonnes of clothing imported into the UK every year ends up in our landfills. The really sad thing is that even charity shops have to send high quantities of unsold clothing to landfill, too.

YOUR OWN LOOK

Give yourself a little challenge and ask how much you can reduce your spending on clothes, how much you can reuse what you already have by adapting and accessorizing, and how much you can recycle. Give away what you no longer wear to the charity shop or on Freecycle (this is especially welcome for children's clothes, www.freecycle.org), sell it or, if it's beyond redemption, cut it up and use the fabric to wrap gifts or make cushion covers if it's pretty, or to use for rags and cloths to save on disposable paper kitchen towels.

Apart from the obvious waste and unsustainability of buying cheap 'disposable' high street clothes, the other issue is that everyone else will look the same as you, so why not buy something that's a one-off from an ethical designer? You may only be able to afford one piece rather than three, but it will last far longer and offer you individuality and sustainability. You can mix and match quality items with budget clothes for a great, unique look.

SWISHING

Another great way of sourcing designer outfits is to go 'Swishing' – naff word but great concept. Clothes-swap parties are the new Avon or Tupperware party, and can be a very tiny or a very big affair. It might be an evening in someone's front room – if you're the host then make sure you beg, steal or borrow plenty of dress rails, hangers and full-length mirrors. Have a few screens or areas where people can try clothes on, too, have a couple of bottles of wine (or some de-alcoholized pink fizz – *see the Alcohol chapter*) and make it a fun evening. Or it could be a bigger organized affair in a school hall or even a theatre, where you pay a few pounds to enter, perhaps as a fundraiser, and you get your pick of some wonderful kit. Remember, one girlfriend's castoff can be another's perfect find.

CHARITY SHOP CHIC

I am queen of charity-shop chic, and I'm proud to say I can usually find the gems in charity shops. I think it stems from having had, in my younger days, almost no money but an absolute determination to create my own style. My scrimping and saving has stood me in good stead, I've got some fabulous charity shop finds; the only problem is it becomes quite addictive so I do find myself drawn to charity shops, having a good old rummage even when I don't really need yet another handbag or black jacket – I suppose at least I'm keeping it out of landfill!

Of course one step up from simply rummaging in jumble sales and charity shops is to opt for the vintage look. Most charity shops pick out their proper vintage kit now and add a higher price tag. Do try your find on, though, as women's dress sizes seem to have varied over the years. I bought a fabulous 1950s dress in my usual size, didn't have time to try it on and found it was cut very differently to our fashions. I simply couldn't get it over my shoulders – oh, well, that one got recycled at the next clothes-swap party!

The queen of shopping, Mary Portas, has recently launched her living-and-giving charity shops. The idea is you buy something and hand something back. She's also revamped several rundown charity shops and taught them how to make the best of the vintage finds: www.maryportas.com.

There are dress-exchange shops in many high streets, too. You can take your decent quality items in and they will give you the money if they sell them, minus their commission. Of course the clothes are more expensive than in a charity shop, but you can find some great clothes in excellent condition.

You can also buy from auction sites, of course. eBay has lots of vintage clothing, as does www.myvintage.co.uk. And check out www.bigwardrobe.com.

For everything that's hot about ethical fashion, sign up to the excellent webzine 'Style will save us', at www.stylewillsaveus.com.

VINTAGE FAIRS
There are some great vintage fairs across the UK now:
- www.blindlemonvintage.co.uk
- www.vintagefashionguild.org

REVAMP

Just as clothes-swap events are popping up across the country, there are also lots of initiatives for revamping and restyling vintage clothing. 'Heavenly Anarchist' (www.heavenlyanarchist.com) is one such tiny company which is making a difference. It's basically a couple of people dedicated to creating unique clothing without compromising their ethics. They call their outfits OOAK (one of a kind), all done using eco-friendly fabrics and trims, recycled materials and organics, green energy and eco-friendly detergents in the production. I bought a gorgeous chintzy dress with blue velvet tassels for my little girl; it had clearly been made from curtains – I felt a scene from *The Sound of Music* coming on! Maria – the original recycling queen!

There's a whole industry, too, grown up around alterations. Rather than chucking out something that no longer fits us, we should have it altered or – even more funky – turned into a completely different garment.

For wonderful recycled clothing, you should also check out www.fashion-conscience.com.

HIGH STREET INITIATIVES

Some high street shops now also have a section for original retro kit, and some stock organic cotton clothing, but check the credentials carefully to make sure that the garments are fairly traded. Some stores have signed up now to the Ethical Trading Initiative, and some such as Marks and Spencer have teamed up with agencies such as Oxfam, and for a time were offering incentives to take back unwanted M & S clothes to Oxfam in return for a voucher. TK Maxx do a fine job of keeping unsold clothes from landfill, some of them classic designer pieces. Who cares if it's a garment from last season? (I never did understand that 'kitting out your wardrobe every season' thing, I often wear ancient summer dresses over trousers in winter with a couple of layers on top.)

Don't forget, too, that you can hire clothes, if it's a one-off for a function or party. It works out at a fraction of the cost of what you'd pay for a really special item.

NEW AND GREEN

On the rare occasions I buy myself or my kids something brand new, I do seek out ethical fabrics, not simply because of the green issues but because these fabrics last longer and are so much nicer to wear. Trust me, you haven't really experienced decent quality fabrics until you've tried real organic cotton, natural breathable fibres and handwoven fabrics. It's not all shades of buff and cream either; there are wonderful plant-based colours that are even more vibrant than their synthetic counterparts. See www.ecotextile.com.

'Labour behind the label' is an ethical trade initiative which will trace the whole process to make sure your choices really are sustainable – www.labourbehindthelabel.org.

A good ethical fabric to look out for is bamboo, which is amazingly soft and light yet sun-protective and anti-sweat: I love the sporty wear from Bam www.bambooclothing.co.uk. They also sell the softest scarves imaginable that make cashmere feel like sandpaper!

You can get great hemp clothing, too, as well as accessories, handbags and more from www.hempish.com.

Take a look at www.ethical-fashions.com or check out eco-couture and high-end eco-fashion such as the range created by Aly Hewson and Bono (www.edunonline.com).

It's also hard to beat People Tree for excellent ethical fashions – www.peopletree.co.uk

See also Ciel www.cielshop.co.uk

For casual wear and yoga kit try www.gossypium.co.uk

Adili www.ascensiononline.com

Eco-eco www.eco-eco.co.uk

Spirit of Nature www.spiritofnature.co.uk

And of course Colin Firth's eco-emporium www.eco-age.com

And a wealth of eco-designers at www.diva-stores.com

JEWELLERY

Choosing jewellery that's kind to the earth is another headache. The whole process of mining for gold can pollute, create toxic waste, threaten the health of workers and displace people from their land. Then there's 'conflict' diamonds to consider.

Buying New

If you're buying new jewellery, find out if the jeweller is a member of the Council for Responsible Jewellers, and ask about their ethical policy.

Look at Cred www.credjewellery.com and Green Carat www.greenkarat.com.

Sustainable Jewellery

For sustainable jewellery, look at www.lajewellery.co.uk – they're part of the slow movement and use recycled silver.

Jewellery made from recycled materials is becoming very fashionable. My kids love making painted pasta shell necklaces for me (which is a start), but a great initiative is to gather up all your own bits and bobs of broken jewellery and accessories and see if you're feeling artistic enough to create something new!

Buying Vintage

Again buying vintage is so much more original, and if there's an old ring that used to belong to your granny remember you could always ask a jeweller to resize it and make it all shiny and beautiful again.

For wonderful eco-accessories and jewellery check out www.puredesigncompany.co.uk.

BAGS

For great bags, it goes without saying no girlfriend should be seen with plastic. This is the era of the uber-gorgeous re-useable bag.

- www.onyabags.co.uk
- www.bagsofchange.co.uk
- www.turtlebags.co.uk

For the innovative '20 bags in one' see the Trolley-Dolly www.zpm.com.

If you're a lover of natural baskets, you can't beat the gorgeous Moroccan ones from www.basketbasket.co.uk.

SHOES

Ditch the image of someone slightly grubby wearing sandals with socks; you can get excellent Fairtrade animal-friendly footwear that's hardwearing and stylish. To mention just a few suppliers:

- www.vegshoes.co.uk
- www.freerangers.co.uk 100 per cent vegan shoes

- www.greenshoes.co.uk lovely handmade ethical shoes
- www.hempish.com great shoes made from hemp

There're also some innovative shoes made from recycled materials. I've seen some funky shoes, along with bags of all sizes and designs, made from recycled car tyres. Very bouncy! www.simpleshoes.com and www.lovethoseshoes.com.

MAKE DO AND MEND

It's not that long ago that our mums would have simply darned our socks or added a stitch or two into a blouse that was coming adrift. Fortunately there's been a bit of a shift, and while I'm not sure any of us will ever repair our socks or undies, we are realizing the value of elongating the life of our clothing and revamping something we thought we couldn't wear again.

If, like me, you simply cannot sew (in truth my eyesight is so poor I find it tricky to thread a needle), then cheat and use Velcro, or even glue! My girlfriend who works as a costume assistant in film and TV often suggests turning a boring knee-length but well-fitting skirt into a mini-skirt simply by cutting it and using Copydex glue. Add an edging of funky braid and you have a great new skirt.

'Haberdashery' is a fabulous forgotten word but go seek it out: collect a treasure box of ribbons, braids, threads and buttons and you'll never be without the resources you need to create wonderful garments. Kids love doing this, too, and it gets you out of the hideous expense of needing to buy costumes for them for Halloween – you can sew (or glue) your own pumpkin head or ghostly cloak!

Buttons are the new rock 'n' roll; pick them up at jumble sales and charity shops and if – God forbid – you are going to be throwing away rather than recycling clothes, always cut the buttons off first. Many a boring dress, jacket or coat can be fashioned into something great just by changing the buttons.

DYES

You remember tie-dyeing at school? Well, give it another go, it's a great way to revamp tired discoloured garments and shoes. Of course you don't have to go for the tie-dye look, just turn your white top pink!

Avoid dyes that contain Azo; look for those that are free from toxic chemicals (such as cold-water dyes). You can make your own plant-based natural dyes with wonderful vibrant colours, even from plants in your own garden – ubersustainable!

For recipes, see www.nationalgardenmonth.org.

FABRIC PAINTING

If you're artistic, why keep your creations for the wall? Wear your art – literally.

You can buy fabric paints and fabric pens which will fix well simply by ironing the garment. Craft shops should have non-toxic fabric paints.

KNITTING

This has made a real comeback; there are knitting clubs popping up everywhere and I'm banking on a knitted purse for Christmas courtesy of my nine-year-old. Buy sustainable wool; rather like your foodstuffs, it's a good idea to think local, buying British wool and, wherever possible, from rare breeds to keep their strong genetic line. Excellent British wools such as Merino wool and Cornish wool are beautifully soft.

If you're a fan of good wool and love your woolly socks, check out Corrymoor Socks www.corrymoor.com – SO warm.

LOOKING AFTER YOUR CLOTHES

Undoubtedly your clothes will give you better service if you treat them well. The heap on the floor will not cut it for long, so treat yourself to some decent clothes hangers and make time to care for your clothes. If like me you have a horribly overstuffed wardrobe, then have a big de-clutter and you may find some forgotten gems in the process. For some girls it works to hang all the long items together, then all the shorter ones with shoes underneath. I know they do say put your shoes in boxes and stick a photo of the shoes on the front – good on you if you're that organized, mine are in a heap, sadly, though the one really good pair of killer heel boots are sitting neatly wearing shoe trees. I must confess they look the least battered of my footwear collection. Sort your clothes into colours too if that helps you to see what you have, but whatever you do, hang them up and make time for mending them or altering if they need it.

Dry Cleaning

See the chapter on Home for doing the laundry, but just a quick word here about dry cleaning.

A large number of clothes do come with that scary three-word command *Dry clean only*. I usually avoid buying these, because not only do I not want the cost of regular dry cleaning but I also don't want the carcinogenic chemical residues anywhere near me. I also don't need swathes of plastic and safety pins.

I have it on good authority from my costume designer friend that many garments that say dry clean only, especially if they're natural fabrics, are much better off simply being handwashed at a low temperature or handwashed gently, rinsed in cold water and left to dry flat. This is certainly the case with silk and cashmere. In fact, you will prolong the life of the fabrics this way rather than breaking down the fibres with the harsh chemicals used in dry cleaning.

If you simply must dry clean, then go to a dry cleaner who uses the 'Green Earth' process – it's a silicon-based solvent rather than the really insidious Perc (perchloroethylene) used by the majority. www.greenearth.co.uk

If you've had clothes dry cleaned, always let them air well before putting them back in your wardrobe.

Remember steam cleaning, too (see the Home chapter). A quick blast with a steam cleaner can freshen up a winter coat in no time.

See www.ethicalfashionforum.com for more on ethical fashion, and also see *Eco Chic: The Savvy Shoppers Guide to Ethical Fashion* by Katherine Hamnett and Matilda Lee.

Janey's Guide to Staying Well

I'm going to need to use the word 'holistic' when talking about health. It's not my favourite word, but I genuinely can't think of another one that really does mean 'the whole picture', and when we're talking about health, 'whole' is what we're aiming for.

In addition to some tips and ideas for natural remedies for common ailments, there's a lot in this chapter about the 'body–mind' connection. Without doubt our thoughts and emotions affect our health. If the concept of the 'power of the mind' is new to you, I'll recommend some wonderful further reading on the subject.

It's still commonplace to try to find a 'pill for every ill', but lots of us (happily, 'consciousness' is the new rock 'n' roll) know that in many instances it's impossible to isolate one condition and treat just that. GPs' surgeries are full of the 'worried well' who show up with, say, a backache, chat to the GP for the allotted seven minutes and leave with a prescription for some painkillers and a sick note from work. The enlightened few, and in this instance I use that word advisedly (it is a depressingly small number of girlfriends so far) dig a little bit deeper, asking themselves what is going on. They may ask if they've strained a muscle lifting a child or a heavy object without bending their knees properly, or indeed have something emotional going on – because in many cases pain in the back relates quite literally to not feeling supported. A pain in the neck can literally signify that something or someone needs to be 'removed' from your life. Chest pains (obviously having ruled out serious heart conditions etc) can literally be your body nudging you to consider what it is you need to 'get off your chest'.

I'm very much in Louise Hay's *You Can Heal Your Life* territory here. If you haven't read that life-changing, incredible book, make that your very first task when you put this book down!

I do have first-hand experience of the theory. I am a big fan of long-term breastfeeding. I won't bore you with the details, but I'm patron of the Association of Breastfeeding Mothers, so after managing to breastfeed my first son successfully till he was almost three, I fully expected to do the same with my second baby. The issue was that for a while I was 'tandem feeding' – now, that doesn't mean breastfeeding on a bike, it means feeding two babies at once – and, quite frankly, it takes it out of you!

When my first boy was almost three and weaning himself naturally and my second baby was around 14 months, I started to have all kinds of health issues. I felt knackered (but I figured that was par for the course with two young children). I also felt slightly headachy (again, I put that down to tiredness). But then my body decided to let me know in no uncertain terms that I needed to address something. I got a very painful earache. A weird one; I'd never had earache before (boy, am I sympathetic now to anyone who suffers).

I tried all the natural 'remedies' that I knew worked for others, but nothing seemed to sort it. I went to see a naturopathic nutritionist consultant, who said it was likely my immune system needed a boost. She suggested perhaps all my essential nutrients were being taken away by breast-feeding. I brushed it off, saying, 'Oh no, I've done it before.' The nutritionist didn't push it and it was only when a friend asked me 'Have you read Louise Hay's books? Have you asked yourself the literal question – "Why do I have earache – what could it be that I am not wanting to hear?"' that I realized the answer was clear. I didn't *want* to give up breastfeeding. It made me feel 'needed', and reinforced my own perception of being a 'good mother'. Ultimately, however, my body needed to heal and was giving me the call to action. I weaned my toddler the next day – he didn't seem to care! The earache went away instantly.

I've never forgotten that important lesson. Now whenever I have symptoms I think carefully – where in my body is the problem, what could my body be telling me?

Of course it's not always that simple, and God forbid you think I'm being flippant about serious illness. If any symptoms persist you *must* always seek medical attention. I simply urge you to consider at the same time the 'body–mind' connection.

LET FOOD BE YOUR MEDICINE

Of course, prevention is always better than cure – so how do we ensure that we are as well as we can be? Well, it may not surprise you to know that I'm going to nag you to read, if you haven't read it already, the chapter on food. Yes, gals, when it comes to health and well-being we really are 'what we eat' – and, I would say, what we think.

If you haven't made the connection before, now is the time to get to grips with this really very basic concept. The 'fuel' you provide your body with, both physically and mentally, will 'power' you to optimum health, vitality and well-being or, indeed, low-level dis-ease and ongoing health conditions.

Fancy a night in with a fantastic DVD? My top suggestion is *Food Matters* – though this is one movie where you'd best skip the popcorn and cola. It's essentially a talking heads documentary about nutrition – or the lack of it – in the average Western diet. Most gals when they watch it say that they feel as though the 'light' has literally come on and life is never quite the same again.

The basic message given by the many eminent doctors, investigative journalists and cancer specialists is the same: we need a new paradigm in healthcare across the Western world. What we're doing sure isn't working, and our health is failing because the one thing that could really bring about change isn't being addressed. Doctors and healthcare professionals study pharmaceutical drugs for years, but in most cases get less than a day's training in nutrition. Simple changes – a diet high in organic fruit and veg, the right vitamins and minerals (in cases of deficiency), exercise and stress-reduction – work as both prevention and cure for most disease states. Eating fruit and veg, drinking fresh vegetable juices, taking regular exercise and looking after your mind allows the body to heal itself without the need for medication, which may suppress the symptoms temporarily but also weaken your immune system.

Nutritionist Andrew W Saul, PhD, tells us that treating illnesses as serious as cancer with the right diet and high-dose vitamins has proven incredibly effective, yet the media and medical professionals tell us to 'beware of vitamins, they can be dangerous'. Interestingly, Andrew states that in 23 years of monitoring in the US, only 10 deaths have ever been attributed allegedly to vitamins, and even those are unverified. Meanwhile, in just one year, 106,000 people died in the US from taking properly prescribed prescription drugs.

Closer to home, we should know that approximately 10,000 people die every year from taking prescription medication. These are not people who have been incorrectly diagnosed or who have not followed the instructions on the pill bottles. Read the warnings and contraindications on the labels and you'll see why.

To put these 10,000 cases in perspective, Phillip Day, a UK-based investigative health journalist and director of the Campaign for the Truth in Medicine, asks us to remember that fatalities from car accidents stand at approximately 3,500 yearly, yet we're constantly peddled the message that we should be 'scared' of vitamins and minerals.

On that note, by the way, as we go to print, the EU directive on vitamins and mineral supplements is still being fought by an organization called Consumers for Health Choice. If the battle is lost there will be restrictions in place regarding the strength of vitamins and minerals. For patients seeking a higher dose (many people swear by taking 1,000 mg of vitamin C, for example), that means taking the tablets in greater quantities, which in turn means more sweeteners and fillers, not to mention more cost and packaging to be disposed of. Why? Well, a cynic might say it's because being healthy doesn't make enough money for the pharmaceutical companies!

British journalist Jerome Burne believes it's entirely right and proper that pharmaceutical companies are focused on making profits, not on wellness. He believes in our capitalist system, but he stresses that the problem lies with the fact that the regulators are financed by the very same companies, so their findings may not be as impartial as we'd like.

Please don't get me wrong. I'm not decrying the whole medical profession. There are some incredibly devoted healthcare professionals. I also, of course, accept that some medical intervention will be necessary in many situations. We should rejoice that lives can be saved, we have world-class surgeons and highly effective life-saving drugs, and preparations are in place for emergencies and acute conditions. In my opinion, for just about everything else we should look for a natural solution. Your body can usually heal itself if you nourish it with the right fuel.

Most of us have our cars serviced at least yearly to pass their MOT. In the interim we ensure that we pump the tyres and fill up with the right fuel in order to prevent them breaking down too often. We forget, however to take the same responsibility for our bodies and minds.

PREVENTION IS ALWAYS BETTER THAN CURE

It seems almost too simplistic to say 'Eat the right foods, supplement where necessary, exercise and reduce stress levels and you'll be well,' but nature has provided us with everything we need. A group of Japanese islanders called the Okinawans consistently live to the ripe old age of around 105, and it's documented that in addition to their unstressed, natural and healthy outlook on life, they eat at least ten portions of fruit and veg every day.

Further reading: *The Rainbow Diet and How It Can Help You Beat Cancer* by Chris Woollams.

See the chapter on Food for much more about nutrition, but remember we could live on avocados alone. We wouldn't want to, of course, but they do contain all the essential minerals and essential fats. (They're higher in potassium even than bananas.) You may already know that ginger and garlic are fantastic natural antihistamines, honey is antibacterial, and cherries are proven to help with arthritis and fibromyalgia. A handful of cashew nuts is fantastic for combating depression.

Dark green, leafy veg is extremely high in antioxidants. Interestingly, so are red and purple foods, so have some prunes along with blueberries and red grapes for breakfast and you'll be doing well.

In my kitchen we have a great 'eat the rainbow' wall chart. The kids love ticking off how many of the health-giving coloured foods they've managed to eat that day. I did, however, have to explain that jelly babies don't count!

You can buy your own rainbow food chart, see www.lemonburst.co.uk.

MIND POWER

A well-stocked kitchen cupboard is full of remedies, if we know how to harness them. More on this later; for now, let's talk about the really important bit: your mind. Even with the best food, drink, vitamins and minerals you will not thrive unless your mind is in order. Even conventional doctors now recognize that happy thoughts are essential to the release of healing endorphins.

Let's look at a few factors that will stop your mind from keeping in good shape.

STRESS LEVELS

However healthily you eat and drink, you will not achieve holistic health and well-being if your head is not 'sorted'. I'm pointing a finger at you, high-flying girlfriend, but trust me, three more and a thumb are pointing back at me. I am, or at least used to be, Queen of Stress, Worry and Anxiety. Close friends frequently would say to me, 'Stop worrying – you'll give yourself a heart attack.' I saw a close friend get cancer and have her breast removed; she was the epitome of health but put her own illness down to stress. In my own case I had some hormonal problems and didn't have a menstrual period for over a year. My naturopathic doctor put it down fairly and squarely to stress damaging my adrenals – scary stuff.

We all know that stress is not good – well 'good stress', or perhaps we should call it excitement and anticipation, can be necessary and beneficial, but not constantly. Most of us opt for some kind of tool to help us relax. Perhaps a cigarette, an alcoholic drink or, in my case, coffee. When I was feeling pent-up, having a coffee would seem to help. In reality, aside from my 'addiction mentality', this was fuelling the problem, exacerbating my stress and keeping me in an adrenaline state. You'll know the phrase 'fight or flight' – adrenaline is all very well when we need to get out of danger, but few of us need to run from tigers these days!

If you are keeping yourself in a low-level stressed state for long periods of time without allowing for proper relaxation and recovery time, here's a way of turning it on its head. Think of the phrase 'fight or flight' literally: when you're feeling stressed over something, why not fly? Not literally (unless you are in fact a secret superhero), but go for a run, a fast walk or anything that will blow the cobwebs away. Get outside whenever you can. Nature has the ability to help us get back in the flow. If possible, take off your shoes and connect with the earth; you'll feel grounded.

Supplements

Remember that your diet will affect your stress levels. Make sure you have an adequate intake of essential fatty acids. We women need good sources of omega 3 oils, so if you're not vegetarian opt for the purest you can find (www.minami-nutrition.co.uk). For veggies, Udo's Choice is a blend of omega 3, 6 and 9 and is great to add to smoothies. I also use flax oil or hemp oil.

You can also buy Cool Oil – a great blend of organic seed oils available in supermarkets. Also try Viridian's Ultimate Beauty Complex Veg Caps www.viridian-nutrition.com. Nuts and seeds are fantastic, too. Keep a bowl of mixed nuts and seeds on hand to snack during the day. For a real treat (not raw, but then I am imperfect!) toast a mix of pumpkin, sunflower and sesame seeds, linseeds and hulled hempseeds with a dash of organic tamari sauce in a hot frying pan, allow to cool and add half a teaspoon of fresh chillis, chopped really fine. You could also try this with just toasted blanched almonds.

For when you need a really healthy snack in a pack, try Conscious Foods handmade, unrefined gluten-, dairy- and wheat-free power snacks: www.consciousfood.co.uk.

Girlfriends' Natural Secrets . . . *Diet wise – don't be afraid of raw, fresh oils and fats – they are what the body needs for nerves, skin and hormones. It is the cooked and heated fats which are the toxic, fattening ones.*

Use a face mask of mashed avocado, powdered spirulina or wheatgrass powder mixed to the right consistency with a little rose water or filtered water – a great nourisher and skin food. Use this once a fortnight to feed and nourish the skin.

– Dr Enid Taylor, colonics and nutritional therapist

Vitamins

B vitamins are also really important for stress levels. I find that when I stop taking them I feel quite 'jittery'. While we're on the subject of vitamins and minerals, I'd say of course in an ideal world we'd get everything we need from our immaculate, healthy diet, but sadly that's not the reality for many of us. Even if we were pretty wholesome, ditched all processed foods and stimulants and ate the right amount of fresh fruits, veg, nuts and seeds, it's still likely we'd need supplementation due to the depletion of minerals and nutrients in our soil and the processes used in modern farming, which contribute to the depletion of the vitamins and minerals in our foods.

In addition to the aforementioned essential fatty acids and B vitamins, I highly recommend that women take vitamin C and perhaps a good-quality multi-vitamin. It's highly likely that at certain times many of us will also need extra calcium and magnesium, selenium and zinc. We've already mentioned the importance of vitamin D; it's thought that, unless you're able to achieve some time in the sunshine every day, you may need to take a supplement – so the list goes on!

It can be incredibly confusing walking into a health store and seeing a whole wall of vitamins and minerals. The best way to determine your individual needs is to see a good nutritionist or naturopathic practitioner. There are also some wonderful high-tech diagnostic tools such as the Vega machine and the excellent Asyra system (www.asyra.co.uk). It's a great way to determine what your body needs nutritionally.

Your diet will be the key to staying young. Marilyn Glenville has this to say about looking great as you age.

Staying Young Naturally

'There's no need to accept that weight gain, wrinkles, dry skin and a whole host of other problems are inevitable aspects of ageing. One way you can combat the wear-and-tear factor is by stalling the action of free radicals on your body. These highly reactive compounds are produced during your body's normal metabolic processes, and also by such things as air pollution and overheating certain oils. They can attack and damage the genetic code and memory of your cells.

'Rust is a product of oxidation, triggered by free radicals. What about wrinkles? Free radicals are the culprits

of those, too. They also contribute to cancer and heart disease.

'You can't do anything to prevent free radicals, but your body does have defence mechanisms that can clear them away.

'A healthy diet is your front line of defence. All vegetables are longevity foods, but perhaps the ones with the most power to prevent premature ageing are broccoli, Brussels sprouts and kale. Leafy greens are loaded with nutrients that can help to prevent free-radical attack.

'Nutrients called antioxidants – vitamins A, C and E, as well as zinc and selenium – are the key players in an anti-ageing diet. Found in vegetables, nuts and fruits, antioxidants are your body's defence against free-radical attack. Make sure you eat a rainbow of fruits and vegetables, for example, leafy green vegetables, berries, carrots and beetroot.

> – Dr Marilyn Glenville, nutritionist specializing in women's health: www.marilynglenville.com

ALLERGIES

If you know or suspect that allergies are a problem for you, try a diagnostic session with a health kinesiologist. They are my number-one choice for sorting problems including emotional issues with children: www.health4health.org.uk.

Also look into some non-allergenic alternatives to common household items such as bedding, and consider some ionizers to refresh the air.

See www.allergybestbuys.com. Also try EFT (Emotional Freedom Technique) www.emofree.com. It has great results with some allergic reactions.

FEELING SAD?

Remember, too, the importance of light. It's been found that 86 per cent of patients suffering from seasonal affective disorder (SAD) will respond to bright light, but you don't have to be a SAD sufferer to benefit from 'seeing the light'. First, get out into daylight every single day. If you or someone you know is anxious or depressed, encourage them to take a brisk walk every day.

Get yourself a light box. They have achieved incredible results for people who aren't serious sufferers by having the light on near to where they're working, eating or pottering for just 20 minutes a day. See the chapter on Home (page 249) for more about this.

RELAX AND REJUVENATE

Most of us – me included – are so caught up with our never-ending 'to do' lists we don't stop to really rejuvenate ourselves, yet we all know, deep down, how much easier it is to function, how much more patience and tolerance we have, how much happier we are when we've had some recreation time. I try to remind myself that I need to 'recreate' myself, putting all the bits back together rather than being that stressed-out fragmented bundle of nerves.

MEDITATION

Meditation is undoubtedly one of the best ways of clearing the mind and experiencing total relaxation. People who meditate regularly, even for only 20 minutes a day, say that they feel the benefits in every area of life. If only it weren't so goddamn hard! If you're anything like me, as you sit trying to meditate a thousand things come into your mind. After many years I finally hit upon a way that works for me. I now make sure I'm comfortable, sit straight and listen to a CD of alpha waves, produced as part of a healing programme called The Alpha Matrix – see page 123 for more on this.

As you drift off to sleep, you can also listen to one of the healing programmes from Innertalk www.innertalk.co.uk. They claim great results in everything from reducing stress to increasing your bust size!

I also try and have a few minutes in every hour that are designated for rejuvenation. If you can't do some simple stretches or have a quick walk in the fresh air, then phone a girlfriend. Make sure it's someone who lifts your spirits, not drains your energy. Even just close your eyes and go in your mind to your 'special place'. To assist any relaxation it's a great idea to have a place to go in your head. Make it some-where you love: the beach, your garden, perhaps a meadow or a waterfall. Make sure you can envision it in great detail, the colours, the sounds, the smells. For me, if I'm having a stressful day, a few minutes once an hour 'going off' to my favourite beach in St Ives does the trick.

MINDFULNESS

I also now practise mindfulness. There are numerous books on this and I highly recommend you read one: *The Mindful Way Through Depression: Freeing Yourself from Chronic Un-happiness* (includes Guided Meditation Practices CD) by Mark Williams, John Teasdale, Zindel Segal and Jon Kabat-Zinn is great and you don't need to consider yourself seri-ously depressed to benefit. There's also the classic *Grist for the Mill* by Ram Dass.

If you're thinking, 'Oh, I'm simply too frantic,' that used to be me, too. I was always such a jittery, busy person I didn't really get the 'still your mind' thing. For me the most useful advice was simply to acknowledge while meditating or relaxing that thoughts are coming into my mind, notice them and let them go.

You can practise mindfulness in many ways, but the simplest is just to acknowledge the 'now'. It can be as simple as going for a walk and noticing the sounds you hear, the sights you see, how you are feeling, but keep your thoughts in the present, the here and now. As soon as your mind wanders off to the invitations you need to send out for your little girl's party, or what ingredients you need for the cake you're going to bake, then accept and acknowledge that you are slipping into 'planning' mode. If you find yourself reliving events of the day, accept that you are in 'remembering' mode. Get back to the present. Most of us spend large parts of our day and life planning and getting stressed about the future, yet the only absolute certainty is the moment we're in now and we should all strive to be fully living in it.

There are many ways to include mindfulness in your daily life. Remember that as humans we need constant change, so make little changes in your routine. Take a different route to work, try a new exercise class, try a new juice or smoothie. When you get dressed in the morning choose something that lifts your spirits when you look at it, even a scarf or a piece of jewellery will do the trick. Remember the importance of scent, too – see The Power of Fragrance chapter.

THE POWER OF PRAYER

Prayer works, there's no doubt. In times of crisis most people will pray just in case there's a God or higher power, even if they've never considered it before. If you want to try prayer, don't worry about needing to be in church or on your hands and knees. Anywhere, anytime will do. Some people find they feel really connected to their higher self if they go and soak up the atmosphere in an old church or cathedral. When I was going through a bad patch many years ago, I couldn't face going to church and conversing with people, so I just took myself off to St Albans Abbey for their services. I enjoyed being completely anonymous in the huge congregation.

Remember, too, that there's immense power in numbers. If you need love, light and prayer sent to someone you love, then get onto your social networks and ask for support. Ask everyone to send love at a specific time.

I had my own taste of this just recently when a friend's ten-year-old son who has a serious medical condition was suddenly rushed to a hospital and was in a coma. A whole group of us chose a time and decided to send him love, light, prayers, energy, healing – whatever. I asked everyone on my Facebook fanpage and forum to join us and got an overwhelming positive response back. In truth, as my family and I lit a candle at 7.15 that night and sent all our combined healing thoughts to this boy, I felt I was going through the motions, not really expecting anything to change. Imagine my sheer joy, then, when I heard he woke fleetingly at 7.30 p.m. Three days later he was recovering at home, seemingly unscathed by his ordeal. Doctors used the word 'miracle'. Coincidence? We'll never know. Force of numbers is powerful stuff – mountains have been moved!

HEALING YOUR MIND

There are so many different types of healing for the mind that it's impossible to list them all here. We are blessed now with so many healers who have a genuine gift, I can only tell you of my experiences and suggest that you get recommended to a good healer, coach or counsellor.

Can you look better and sort your stress simultaneously? Tej Semani is one of the world's leading sports and education psychologists, and a cognitive behavioural specialist. I visited him when my stress levels were off the scale, as I'd heard he had developed a treatment that uses brainwave technology for holistic healing and well-being. You may be familiar with Alpha Healing, but Tej's therapy is about combining psychological treatment with cognitive therapy – which involves keeping your brainwaves at a certain frequency through listening to specific sounds and frequencies. The premise is that you can 'retune' your brainwaves and maintain a positive state of mind.

It works on the premise that the better you feel on the inside the better you will look on the outside. Tej's surgeon colleague has noted time and again that those with a good state of mind heal faster from all types of surgery. This 'auric' brain training works brilliantly on migraines, sleep disorders and stress and, as someone who has suffered from fairly severe stress, I must say it is very effective. In short, Tej helped me in a very short space of time to focus on my priorities, helped me find a plan of action and gave me the all-important Alpha Healing tracks to play whenever I needed a boost.

I've asked Tej if we can easily sort out our stress. Here is his answer:

'None of us was born stressed, in fact it is said that we learn how to feel "stressed out" properly when we hit our teens (in today's age it is getting much younger). Stress is

what we call in psychology a "learned response", and if you learn something you can most definitely unlearn it.

'What does "unlearning" stress actually mean? For starters, the secret to a happy life is to be in control of how you react to and feel towards situations. Life is a process of opposites: Good and Bad, Love and Hate, Peace and Frustration come together as pairs, you cannot have the positivity of one without experiencing the negativity of the other from time to time. When you know that it is OK to not feel good all the time, you reach a stage of understanding that leads to being in control of how you feel towards a situation, empowering you to prevent the negativity of the stressful situation from overwhelming you.

'The key place to be within yourself is in a place of balance, what sports professionals call being "in the zone" – that is, in a state of mind where you will not be negatively affected by situations that previously would have caused stress. Psychologically we are at our best and happiest when the balance and order in our lives outweighs the uncertainty and chaos, when we can take a situation which can easily cause stress and approach it with a sense of detachment.

Step 1: Awareness
'View any initial twinges or early onsets of stress as a signal. Take a physical step back from any stress you're experiencing, and acknowledge to yourself that this situation may cause your stress (yes, it is that simple for the first step).'

Step 2: Detachment

'Detach yourself from the situation and tell yourself to remain in the present moment, rather than dwelling on something that's happened in the past or worrying about something that hasn't happened in the future. A good and quick way to stay in the present is to place your attention on your core (around your tummy) and take three deep breaths. Try it now and notice immediately how quickly your attention comes back to this present moment.'

Step 3: Balance

'Your next step is to focus on how you want to feel. Ask yourself the following question:

"If I could choose to feel anyway I could, what would I choose?" Say if it's calm or relaxed, think of something (it can be anything in that moment) that relaxes you or calms you. Focus on that and you will find your stress, anxiety levels decrease right away.'

Step 4: Gratitude

'Every day, focus for a few minutes on three people or things in your life which you are grateful for. The act of being grateful is so vital for our ongoing emotional and physical health and well-being, but it is a choice. You can choose to let a situation overwhelm you or you can ignore certain aspects of a situation and eventually become numb or you can move through an event and eventually reach a place where you say, "Hey, I learned something here." Then the next time a stressful situation hits you, you are armed not only with knowledge, but a

neurological and physical resilience that is the result of the previous decision you made on focusing on what you want to feel.'

– Tej Samani, Cognitive Behavioural Specialist
www.the-alpha-matrix.com
www.theunlearningfoundation.com

STILLNESS BUDDY

For a quick fix at your computer, this is such a simple idea. It is a software application called Stillness Buddy. It helps people to remain mindful of the present moment, relaxed and at peace, while working at the computer. It works by displaying short 'moments of stillness' and longer 'mindfulness pauses', interspersed throughout the day.

The great news is that the breaks are designed to be very brief, so they don't interfere with work or other commitments. You can choose the duration and frequency to suit your preferences and schedule. I've found it really effective – well, like right now while I'm beavering away writing I just need to take a few moments out, so the Stillness Buddy can help me to focus on taking a few moments out rather than letting my mind wander off onto the fact that the washing needs doing …

You can find more about the Stillness Buddy and download a free 30-day trial, at www.stillnessbuddy.com.

SHAMANIC HEALING

I had no real expectations when I first went for shamanic healing. My healer, Dawn Paul, seemed really quite – well, 'normal'. I suppose I was expecting someone from an Inca tribe using smoke and feathers rather than a tall glamorous woman living in a modest house in Hertfordshire. I'd heard that shamanic healing was incredibly successful for all manner of ills, and works on both an emotional and physical level. Indeed, without making false claims of miracle cures, it seems Dawn has indeed affected the 'cure' of many people from babies to the elderly from all around the world with conditions as diverse as post-traumatic stress disorder through to cancer and clinical depression.

I went to see her primarily because of hormonal issues, but in addition to talking to me about physical symptoms, much of what she did on that first session was to try to tap into where I was mentally. She uses biofeedback techniques and some 'shamanic cards' to determine which priorities to address. She calls it an energetic assessment.

Shamanic healing is very gentle, yet it works very deeply. We all exist on many different levels – physical, emotional, energetic, mental and spiritual – and we need to be healed on *all* of those levels. Shamanism can sometimes be misunderstood as dark or spooky, but this is not the case at all. Basically, shamanism is around 40,000 years old, and was the medicine of the first peoples of the Earth.

Is it akin to therapy? Well, sort of; I've had counselling and indeed I've had friends who've seen counsellors for 20 years and, despite gruelling sessions of dragging up old memories, have achieved little or no positive result. For me, shamanism seemed to work pretty quickly on the core issues.

Soul Retrieval

Dawn explained to me the concept of *soul retrieval*. She believes soul loss can occur sometimes as a form of protective mechanism after severe emotional, mental or physical shock. She uses an excellent analogy to explain this. She asked me to imagine a Terry's Chocolate Orange, all those segments connected to each other in the foil wrapper. Imagine that the foil wrapper is the body and the segments are the soul. The effects of soul loss on the person will range from depression and low energy to problems with the immune system, poor energy protection and problems finding their place and purpose in the world. In short, they will feel that something is missing, because something *is* missing: those aspects of the soul. Often when people go on a 'big search' – perhaps for the perfect job/partner/purpose in life/spiritual path, etc., what they are actually looking for is those soul parts, those aspects of themselves.

The experience as a whole was profound. During the first session she asked me to lie down while she took me on a guided visualization to connect with my 'inner child'. Yes, she does use smoke and feathers, but trust me this is no hippy charlatan at work. I genuinely feel like I have uncovered deep layers, but better still she has helped me to heal them, and all in two sessions. I can honestly say that in the style of that 'chocolate orange', I feel that my segments are intact!

Here's Dawn's personal take on looking great naturally:

'I am constantly amazed by the changes in clients after a healing session, in fact I have often thought about taking "before" and "after" photos! Holding on to emotional baggage, old wounds, anger, resentment, guilt or pain clogs up our energy field, literally weighing us down and reducing our level of vitality. This affects our immune

system and each cell of our body, and rapidly accelerates the ageing process.

'When I work with clients and enable them to drop a lifetime of emotional baggage, they often look 10 years younger. I can see the changes occurring in their faces as I am working with them! They look fresher, lighter and more energized – and the good news is they feel it, too!

'Getting out in nature has to be the next most important step. We spend more time inside than we should. A scientist named Schumann has discovered that the Earth "hums" at a very low frequency of 7.83 Hz (known as a Schumann Resonance) and this hum is very healing and balancing for the body. So it is not only the fresh air and the exercise that does us good when we are outside, but also the vibration of the Earth herself. Walking on the Earth is good, but lying on it is even better. Just remember to take a blanket with you!

'For easing away those worry lines, nothing can beat meditation! I practised Transcendental Meditation for years and found it highly beneficial in many ways, although any simple meditation will help you. Interestingly, after about 10 minutes I could feel all the tensions draining from my face and all of the muscles releasing, particularly between my eyebrows. These muscle tensions are what cause wrinkles, and no amount of face cream can get rid of them. Meditation is better than Botox! And everyone can do it! Just sit upright, relaxed, and concentrate on breathing into your tummy. As soon as you realize your mind has wandered off somewhere, bring your attention back to your breathing. Do this *for at least 10 minutes and try to build up to 20. You will soon feel the tensions in your face and body start to disappear!*

'Next on the list is loving yourself! So many people are horrible to themselves and this can cause a lot of stress in the body and can show on the face. Treat yourself as if you are your dearest lover! You're worth it! Beauty on the inside, beauty on the outside! And when we love ourselves, that love goes out into the world and we attract love back to us. Can't be bad! Try it!'

— *Dawn Paul www.liberate-online.co.uk*

TREATING YOUR BODY

There are a myriad of therapeutic treatments available to us now, and I'm guessing you already have your favourites. I think it's important, though, to distinguish between 'pampering' such as facials, manicures and pedicures and the healing therapeutic treatments. Don't get me wrong, I am certainly not averse to a facial (I opt for a holistic one using only natural products – Neal's Yard Remedies offer them, and see www.abigailjames.com), and I love having my nails done (seek out a technician willing to work with non-toxic nail polishes – Pure Me in Farringdon and Green Hands in Leominster are two examples). It's lovely to be pampered, but for genuine 'healing' always choose a holistic therapeutic treatment with a really intuitive therapist. I'm going to list a few of my personal favourites here, some more unusual than others!

I have found great benefits from tried-and-trusted therapies such as aromatherapy, reflexology, emotional freedom technique (EFT), colour chakra healing, health kinesiology, creative healing, hot stone massage, thalassotherapy and the Bowen technique. I think it's important to find what suits you when it comes to treatments. Many years ago I had the experience of being 'massaged' in what was then called a 'health farm'. It was cold, austere and I felt like a piece of meat on a slab. Fortunately we've come a long way and health resorts now are usually holistic. Therapists need more than just training, and the best ones have intuitive skills and healing hands.

If you're a girlfriend who doesn't 'treat' herself very often, ask around among your friends for what they'd recommend. If money is tight, ask for a voucher for a treatment for your next Christmas or birthday present. Too many girlfriends spend time looking after other people but forgetting about themselves.

For a list of recommended therapists: Federation of Holistic Therapists www.fht.org.uk.

Bowen

I don't need to talk you through most treatments in detail, but I must tell you a bit about the Bowen technique because I profoundly believe it works like a miracle for so many problems. The most obvious thing it helps with is joint pain of any kind, but it also works for hay fever, tinnitus, headaches and depression. Of course you must find the right practitioner, but for most people if Bowen is going to work, it does so within a couple of sessions. It can often alleviate aches, pains and symptoms that have been going on for years and that no other type of treatment has had success with.

It's rather like a very gentle form of acupressure, done fully clothed and, uniquely, after the therapist has done a few 'moves' on your body (it feels rather like a gentle stroking), he or she will leave the room to allow your body to heal itself. At this point you may well wonder if this is a charlatan at work popping off to send a text during your treatment time, but miraculously after one short treatment the problem is often relieved.

Bowen works by aligning the body, so it also helps with the referred pain that can come after an injury. It's particularly effective for all types of back pain. I have friends and neighbours who will tell you that if they hadn't discovered Bowen they would probably be far less mobile, in one case almost certainly wheelchair-bound.

It's suitable for any age and was devised for use on horses, and found to be incredibly effective, so we know there's no 'faith healing' involved!

It's really worth researching Bowen. I wish there were Bowen A & E departments because often if you get a minor injury, neck pain or a sudden twisted shoulder it would be incredibly beneficial to be able to get it sorted there and then.

Look at www.bowentechnique.com to find a good practitioner. If you're a therapist yourself you may want to consider adding Bowen to your skills. I've often thought I should learn some just to be able to sort out acute problems with the children. Excellent practitioner Jo Lunn has clinics in Worcestershire and London and runs training sessions as well: www.jolunn.co.uk.

Qi Energy Treatments

You may have read the news reports about 'burping monks' in Harley Street a while back, but the Qi energy treatment offered by the Innersound Foundation is certainly no joke. The Chunsoo Qi treatment, which originated in Korea, is a unique combination of acupressure and sound healing to boost the body's energy and restore immunity and vitality. Remarkably, it takes only around 15 minutes for a full body session. I turned up for my first appointment with Master Oh (who certainly has a great aura) at the wonderfully tranquil centre just off Harley Street. The treatment is done fully clothed and is quite hard to describe, save to say that Master Oh uses fairly firm massage techniques on the pressure points while also using sounds resonating from deep in his energy centre. It sounds like a powerful expulsion of breath and at least one sequence during the treatment honestly did sound like a belch!

Qi energy is based on the principle that, due to both environmental degradation and a build-up of negative emotions, many of us simply can't gather enough energy from nature and consequently have blockages which result in low immunity and chronic health problems, including, in some cases, stress, anxiety and depression. It's said to work on a core level, removing toxins from the body, restoring good energy and stabilizing the circulatory system.

I can't pretend that it wasn't painful. As Master Oh was burping, breathing and massaging me, he pressed his fingers quite deep into my abdomen and around my neck, but interestingly as I left the building 20 minutes later I realized that my shoulders and neck felt more relaxed than they had done in a long time. They claim that Qi treatment can help with stress, insomnia, anxiety, migraine, allergies, digestive disorders and hormonal problems. If you can afford a trip to London, it's worth giving this extraordinary treatment a try. Inner Sound Foundation: www.ins-f.org.

Girlfriends' Natural Secrets . . . *I have short treatments on a FAR infrared machine regularly to detox, relax and reduce cellulite!*
— **Sue Donnelly www.integralnutrition.co.uk**

THE IMPORTANCE OF SLEEP

Sleep is hugely important to staying well – interestingly, though, we can be in danger sometimes of making too big a deal of 'sleeping through the night'. There are other cultures where a full eight hours' sleep is not heralded as the Holy Grail. In *The Continuum Concept* by the anthropologist Jean Leidloff, she talks about the Yequana tribe. When members of this tribe are away working together, they sleep together in one room, and it's not unusual for one to wake the others to tell them a joke. They all laugh and then go back off to sleep!

I'm sure you know most of the tricks for getting to sleep. Try lavender oil on your pillow, make sure you do something relaxing before you go to bed, forget watching the news or even reading, if it's a thriller you're engrossed in, calm your mind by listening to relaxing music. If you're into it, classical music has the best calming effect, but make sure it's something you like. For me, relaxation CDs work well and I usually fall asleep before the CD player switches itself off.

As mentioned, try the Innertalk series www.innertalk.co.uk.

You could also try the cold feet approach. If you can, get outside and walk in bare feet on the grass before bed. If that's not realistic, then pop on some wet socks covered by a dry pair. Sounds ridiculous, doesn't it? But it's said to work!

If you want help in the form of a pill, don't think about sleeping pills, they can become addictive. Certain foods are sleep-inducing; these include bananas, lettuce and, if you eat meat, try turkey. Chamomile tea is relaxing, as is green tea (make sure you opt for a caffeine-free green tea, though).

There are many natural remedies for sleeplessness. The herbs valerian and passiflora can be bought in tablet form, and there's an excellent natural melatonin called asphalia, designed to help protect you against electromagnetic pollution with the rather wonderful side effect of helping with sleep: www.asphalia.co.uk.

Weleda also make an excellent sleep remedy called Avena Sativa Comp Drops. For a real double whammy, I thoroughly recommend a bath with Weleda's Lavender Relaxing Bath Milk followed by a few drops of Avena on retiring to bed – it is a miracle combination! My mum has had sleep problems for many years but managed a great night's sleep after trying this. See the chapter on the Home for sleep 'conditions' (how you position your bed and what else is in there have an impact on sleep quality).

HOUSEHOLD REMEDIES FOR COMMON AILMENTS

I hope that reading this will have a big effect on your trips to the pharmacist. I'm hoping you'll almost never need to darken their door. Of course modern medications are fantastic when essential, but for most common complaints nature has provided everything we need, most of it to be found in any well-stocked kitchen cupboard. It's a topic well covered in my other books, so I'll just mention some of the most common problems and suggest a remedy. Often I simply suggest upping various things in your diet (usually involving juice!); this is because I genuinely believe that, given the right environment and the right 'fuel', your body will heal itself of most minor ailments.

Cystitis

You know this, but I'm going to reiterate that if this painful, miserable condition strikes the best thing you can do is take to your bed with a hot water bottle and drink copious amounts of water, avoid all sugar, processed foods and fruit sugars for a day or so, and stick with green, leafy veg, apricots, garlic and small amounts of protein. Asparagus is also very alkalizing, so treat yourself to asparagus soup.

In the chapter on Food I talk about kefir. It's claimed to have many health benefits, from helping to cure constipation to solving all manner of digestive problems, but perhaps its finest hour comes because it contains a yeast called *Candida kefyr* – this is a natural antagonist to *Candida albicans* (the digestive bacteria that, left unchecked, causes thrush), so it can often help with cystitis. Uses include dipping tampons into the kefir and inserting to soothe and clear up vaginal thrush or stop an attack of cystitis as it starts. You can also take probiotics or use a probiotic capsule as a vaginal pessary.

You'll also know about using cranberry juice to help with cystitis. Be careful, though: most regular brands are sweetened and the sugar will not be beneficial at all. If you get the real thing, you'll need to sweeten it with honey or agave syrup.

Period Pains

Herbs can be very effective here:

- Belladonna 30C – for heavy blood loss
- Mag phos 30C – for cramping pains
- Agnus castus – very effective for heavy periods

Of course, evening primrose oil is said to be beneficial in easing premenstrual symptoms. I think if it's possible to see a qualified homeopath, herbalist or nutritionist it will be easier to determine which remedies might work best for you, as symptoms vary so much in hormonal conditions.

Magnetic bracelets can have a great effect on reducing pain. Get the ones that use the same technology as in hospitals (based on central reverse polarity). See www.ecoflow.com. Ladycare also make little magnets that clip onto your knickers, very discreet, and some people find they help alleviate premenstrual cramps. You may also find that replacing tampons with a Mooncup has a dramatic effect on your well-being before your period (see page 163).

Menopausal Symptoms

It won't surprise you to know I don't like the idea of hormone replacement therapy. I'm not there yet, so we'll see if I change my mind if the night sweats and the mood swings start, but I've heard that the herb black cohosh achieves great results, as does *Peuraria mirifica* – an oestrogenic herb which is excellent for menopausal and perimenopausal women. There is a caution to sound, though: *Peuraria* can enlarge the breasts, so if you suspect you could already be oestrogen-dominant, then avoid. Again, see a holistic nutritionist if possible for a more personalized assessment.

It's definitely a good idea to up your intake of essential fatty acids. You can find recipes online for yummy health-giving treats such as hormone replacement cake, which can be made by replacing half the amount of regular flour with soya flour and adding oats, linseed, sesame seeds, almonds and stem ginger.

Colds and Flu

The naturopathic view is that colds, coughs and flu are all part of the body's elimination detoxification process, so a couple of colds a year may not be so terrible. If you find, though, as I did at one time, that you're getting cold after cold and feeling generally rundown, it's time to try and strengthen your immunity. Consider taking some nutritional supplements and schedule in relaxation time for yourself, perhaps a regular massage – and as you relax literally visualize your white blood cells multiplying ready to fight any intruders that come their way.

It's a good idea to steam in, literally, as soon as you feel a cold coming on. Steam inhalation is fantastic for colds and any respiratory problems. Let your head hover about 12 inches from a bowl of boiling hot water to which you've added a few drops of eucalyptus oil or, even better, some crushed eucalyptus leaves. You could also use peppermint tea as an infusion. Drape a towel over your head and inhale, it's a fantastic decongestant and you get a free facial, too. For children, a much safer option is to make a kind of tent by draping a blanket over some chairs, and sit in there with them – it's usually lots of fun – remembering to ensure that the bowl of hot water is out of harm's reach.

Take extra vitamin C, zinc and echinacea for a few days. Homeopathic remedies that can help nip colds in the bud include Aconite 30C and Allium Cepa 6C, especially if you have a streaming nose and watery eyes. It's also definitely worth trying the *Ginger Shot* (see Juicing, page 200), and of course you can make your own ginger tea: grate fresh ginger into a pan of boiling water, then add lemon juice and honey to taste. If you're not expecting too much French kissing, add some garlic to a smoothie. Yes, you'll stink, but it will sort the cold out!

Get as much rest as possible, and try heating up your body. If you can get to a sauna you'll really feel the benefit, or have a hot bath to raise your body temperature. I used to recommend Epsom salts but now feel they can be quite drying (and you should never use if you have high blood pressure or diabetes). Dead Sea salts are good, Himalayan salt is even better, though it can be expensive. After your hot bath, dry off well, wrap up really warm and go to bed with a hot water bottle and a few drops of lavender oil on your pillow.

Girlfriends' Natural Secrets . . . When I was a teen, I experimented with oat bran, cucumber, honey and yoghurt on my skin. I even tried sulphur, as it was meant to give me a light porcelain complexion. Quite difficult to achieve when my skin was the colour of rich caramel. Now I am 41 and wrinkle-free – not due to daubing my face with the contents of my kitchen, but possibly due to not drinking, smoking, a vegetarian diet and being happy. I even got asked for ID last week when I went to buy a kitchen knife, so I guess I must be doing something right.

Girlfriends' Aspirations . . . To put on a West End show that takes children out of this world and into their imagination. It sounds an impossible dream, but I do believe we can make the impossible, possible.

– Marneta Viegas, founder Relax Kids

Coughs and Sore Throats

All the usual suspects are worth trying here. Honey and lemon is soothing. Sage is very good for sore throats, as is Propolis extract. My favourite old-fashioned cough remedy is simply to leave an onion coated in brown sugar overnight; the 'syrup' left behind is very soothing – add some honey to sweeten the slightly bitter taste.

Honey is great generally, of course, and if you can afford manuka honey it's worth taking a teaspoonful with crushed garlic (the taste of the honey overwhelms the garlic).

Hay Fever

And talking of honey, do you know the honey theory? Start taking local honey to desensitize yourself to local pollens as early as possible, around February. I'm sure you know the usual stuff, too, about covering up and using a protective barrier such as the Haymax balm found in health shops (or at www.haymax.biz). The other thing that works a treat for hay fever is regular ginger shots (see Juice section, page 205).

Headaches

First off, drink copious amounts of water – sounds too simple but it really helps!

Feverfew is an excellent remedy for headaches. It's worth getting the capsules from health stores, but chamomile does a similar job, so drink chamomile tea or an infusion of valerian or ginger tea. You could try willowbark, the natural remedy for headaches which aspirin is based on, sold in health stores.

Try a gentle massage too: use small circular movements all around your temples and around the sinuses, and above and below your eyes. You can massage using a few drops of lavender oil or peppermint oil in a base oil around your temples, or apply a tiny amount of tigerbalm (but don't use the petrochemical ones!).

Mouth Ulcers

Often these are a sign of a deficiency, so check that you are getting enough vitamin C and also B vitamins. Make up a tincture with myrrh oil and use as a mouthwash.

Earache

I used to think Hopi ear candles were, quite frankly, daft, but having tried them when I had a mild earache I've changed my view. I now think the treatment's amazing, very relaxing, gentle and easy to do. You look mighty silly lying there with a large cone around your ear and a candle sticking out, but who cares if it solves the problem? You can buy good Hopi ear candles from www.hypnosisaudio.com, or see a therapist.

Also, warmed olive oil dropped gently into the ear, or a massage oil with almond and a few drops of chamomile to massage all around the ear, can work a treat.

Verrucas and Warts

Apply neat tea tree oil, it really works. Garlic is also good.

My son's verruca went after two applications of banana skin – yep, just the inside of the banana skin against the verruca and cover with a plaster. You look a bit mad going to bed like that, but again, who cares if it works?!

Upset Stomach

It's always best where possible to let nature take its course and let your body rid itself of toxins. Whether it's a self-inflicted attack from overdosing on alcohol and rich foods or an attack of food poisoning, it's best to fast and give your system time to recover. Make sure you drink plenty of fluids, though. Peppermint tea is good for digestion. If possible get fresh mint leaves and infuse.

You can boil up fresh ginger with lemon for a really therapeutic drink. Liquorice is said to be great for digestive upsets, too, but obviously not the regular stuff with sugar!

If you suffer from IBS, heartburn or indigestion try aloe vera juice.

If you're vomiting you may need to replace the body's electrolytes, so have a pinch of Himalayan salt in water and eat a banana or avocado if you can for their potassium content. Avoid the commercial sachets of electrolytes if they contain flavourings or artificial sweeteners. If IBS is the problem, take a daily probiotic or kefir (see page 210) and consider having regular colonics.

Hangover

If you've read the chapter on alcohol you may never need this advice again, but in case you overdo it – the solution is to drink water and then some more. Drink before you go out, drink one glass of water for every alcoholic drink and then drink copious amounts of water before going to bed. Take milk thistle tablets before you go out on the razzle too. Before going to bed, take 1,000 mg of vitamin C in water with some honey dissolved in it.

You may want to make up a refreshing essential oil blend if you're feeling dodgy the next day:

- 5 drops grapefruit
- 3 drops rosemary
- 2 drops fennel
- 2 drops juniper

You can inhale the mix, put a little in the bath or, if you want to use it for massage or just to rub along your wrists, then put it into a base oil such as jojoba or almond.

Minor Burns and Wounds

It's annoying, isn't it, but we've all been there, trying to lift a pan from the oven and catching your exposed arm (another great reason to go more raw!). If you have a minor burn, by far the quickest and most effective treatment is to apply aloe vera gel straight from the plant (it works for sunburn or sores, too). The other great tip is to apply neat lavender oil.

- For minor cuts try calendula and hypericum cream.
- Dilute a few drops of tree oil in pure water and apply as an antiseptic.

Honey

For minor wounds you will never go wrong with honey applied topically. As mentioned, manuka honey comes into its own here. Buy the one with the highest 'activity rating' that you can afford. Manuka honey is from very happy bees in New Zealand. All honey has healing properties, though, and many medicinal uses, from minor cuts to ulcerated legs. For more information on its incredible successes see www.apitherapy.biz.

Splinters

Sounds daft, but for tricky cases where it's hard to remove the offending splinter, tape a tiny piece of bread to the splinter with a sticking plaster. The yeast draws out the splinter!

Bites and Stings/Irritated, Inflamed Skin

Try a hydrosol spray of Roman chamomile oil and helichrysum to provide natural anti-inflammatory relief. Make your own or buy Instant Relief Spray from the Sensitive Skincare Company (www.sensitiveskincareco.com).

To replace the cream that a pharmacist prescribes for irritated skin and rashes, try the Ecz-Easy Soothing Balm from Inlight containing olive oil, evening primrose and black cumin (www.inlight-online.com).

Remember, too, that porridge oats in a little bag or sock can be used to alleviate itchy skin (see Skincare page 13).

Girlfriends' Natural Secrets . . . A great body scrub can be made from caster sugar and oil (olive or coconut). I mix the two to make quite a thick consistency — more sugar than oil. This somehow seems to really help my eczema and gets rid of any dry skin. I always use a good moisturizer afterwards or simply some coconut oil. Works wonders. I keep it in a glass jar with a clip lid and good seal and leave it by the bath. Sometimes I'll add some essential oil, usually lavender.

Girlfriends' Aspirations . . . *I would really love to learn to speak Spanish fluently and hope that my daughter, who is currently just one year old, will also learn Spanish.*

– Vicky Willingham

Bruises

- Arnica 30C for soft tissue
- Bellis Perennis 30C for deep tissue areas

You can also apply arnica cream or gel. You can also apply arnica or comfrey cream and make a compress with vinegar. For severe bruises warmed cabbage leaves work

YOUR NATURAL 'MEDICINE' CUPBOARD

In addition to the foodstuffs, honey, garlic, ginger, etc., make sure you have at least the essential oils listed in the chapter on The Power of Fragrance. It's a good idea to have some aloe vera gel or a plant to hand, as well as a selection of teas and herbal tinctures. Stockists include www.baldwins.co.uk and www.hambledonherbs.co.uk.

Flower remedies can be wonderful. Rescue Remedy is very widely used but there are many others that can be concocted to treat subtle moods. My children seem to really respond to them, and love to choose which flowers they need. See www.indigoessences.com for lovely therapeutic essences. For the classic Bach Flower remedies: www.bachcentre.com.

You may also want to keep in stock a small bottle of colloidal silver. It's a mineral solution designed to replenish trace silver, missing in our bodies due to the depletion of soil minerals as a result of modern farming techniques. The silver helps to boost our immune system and gives us natural protection against bacteria and viruses. See www.uk-cs.co.uk.

Homeopathic Remedies

You can buy homeopathic remedies now in high street chemists or from a good homeopathic pharmacist such as Ainsworths (www.ainsworths.com) or Helios (www.helios.co.uk). Both make excellent kits of the most common remedies with a booklet of useful information and suggestions for treating common complaints.

Remember, if symptoms persist, you should *always* consult your health practitioner.

Janey's Guide to Colonics

If you're about to skip this chapter, thinking 'Oh, please, I do NOT want to go there,' trust me, you need to read on.

Only about six months ago I would have said exactly the same. I really thought the kind of people who wax lyrical about enemas and colonic irrigation were at best misguided and at worst barking mad.

I had also heard the scaremongering stories of how unsanitary it can all be, resulting in bowel infections and even worse, and decided it was not for me. So how did I come to be having regular colonics and, indeed, become something of an enthusiast? Fear not, I'm no evangelist for colonics, but if people ask me for my opinion on optimum holistic living (and you sort of have, reading this book), then I simply must tell you of my epiphany in this very sensitive area.

I was introduced to Dr Enid Taylor, a leading naturopath and colonics expert, by a colleague who said, 'You must go and meet Enid and her husband Glenn, she'll give you a thorough nutritional assessment, blood analysis, the works.' What I failed to realize was that 'the works' included my first ever colonic. I felt, quite frankly, rather wimpy about having to say I was scared, so I decided to grin and bear it! Enid explained it all to me clearly and put my mind completely at rest. To cut to the chase, it's not painful. It's a slightly odd sensation, but not one of pain or even discomfort. Basically after the tube has been inserted, warm, sterile and alkalized water is inserted into the lower colon and you're able to lie on your back, head supported and actually view the contents before it's flushed away – quite bizarre and you wouldn't think you'd want to look, but a kind of morbid fascination takes over and as you lie there quite astonished at the size, shape and colour of the waste matter coming through, you can't help but think, 'When might that have come out of my body if I hadn't had this treatment?!'

Often your very first colonic may not produce what the practitioner calls a 'release'; sometimes it takes two or three sessions before you really see the action! In my case I found it to be quite an emotional experience when I finally had the 'release'. It feels rather like a bowel movement – sorry to be so graphic – but I reckon there was literally years' worth of 'stuff' and it brought with it a wave of emotion. That's not uncommon, apparently, and people often cry or laugh as waste matter is finally released. In truth I don't think I realized until I didn't have symptoms anymore that I'd probably had low-level IBS for years. I'd also had a yeast infection. I was given a powder of beneficial bacteria to take after the first colonic to repopulate the 'good guys' in my colon.

After my first colonic my stomach felt quite gripey and uncomfortable for a few days but after the second and subsequent ones (it's recommended that you have a colonic every couple of months after an initial course of three) I felt lighter (well, I *was* lighter – I lost 4 lb in one session) and full of vitality. My skin also looked clearer, which was a great bonus.

You will have used the phrase 'I have a gut feeling'? Well, that's exactly where the feelings are held. Studies show that our cellular memory is held in our gut, the centre of our emotions, so a colonic is not only physically beneficial, sometimes the unexpected bonus is the emotional and spiritual cleansing that goes along with it.

Here's Enid Taylor herself explaining why it's so important:

'Colonic hydrotherapy used to be called colonic irrigation but that can sound like something vaguely agricultural! By removing backed-up toxic waste material, colonic hydrotherapy helps the body to begin to heal itself from things like constipation, IBS, digestive problems and can often be seen in improved skin quality and weight control.

'However, there is more going on than the simple extraction of old waste matter. The massage and conversation (bordering on counselling) from a trained therapist is as valuable as the warm water. Current philosophy is that there is a lot more going on in the gut than mere diges-tion, and books with titles like The Second Brain *and* Gut Instinct *acknowledge that our bowels are almost a metaphor for our mental and emotional lives and a much more active participant in our thinking, feeling and memory. It is often during a heart-to-heart with a colonic therapist, who is gently massaging the vulnerable*

and tender abdominal area, that a personal problem or emotional bottleneck will release and sometimes there are even moist-eyed revelations where private and personal experiences and memories are shared. During this moment, the bowel will often relax and release what it has been holding on to for weeks, months and sometimes years.'

— *Dr Enid Taylor ND, MCMA www.taymount.com*

Try and get a recommendation if you can. Colonic hydrotherapy should always be performed by a trained therapist who has a wide foundation in holistic health; this ensures that adequate emotional support and education on health are available for you as well. It's so much more than a quick treatment to wash out the bowels, and the colonic machines in salons, where the practitioner may not be fully trained, may not be adequate to acknowledge the full potential efficacy of this ancient and wonderful treatment.

Further Reading
Complete Colon Cleanse by Edward Group
Dr Jensen's Guide to Better Bowel Care by Dr Bernard Jensen
Always Look After Number Two by Galina Imrie

Girlfriends' Natural Secrets . . . For beauty and wellness, I love juicing. I juice every morning, lots of green vegetables and an apple. I feel that this puts goodness into your body at the beginning of the day, so that even if you slip up during the course of the day, you have a good reserve. I also have a water distiller, mostly because I think the water tastes better, but I do try to drink plenty of water – at least six glasses a day.

As I sometimes go swimming I noticed my hair had become dry, so I now use virgin coconut oil as a pre-conditioner. I rub it through my hair and leave it for 5 to 10 minutes before I wash it out. It has really made a difference.

The best tonic of all is having a bloody good laugh.

Girlfriends' Aspirations . . . Talking of laughs . . . my aspiration is to have the body of an 18-year-old catwalk model!

– Lynette Tweedale

Janey's Guide to Girly Things

NATURAL SEX

'For God's sake', I hear you cry, 'All sex is "natural"!' Well, yes, but beware the accoutrements! Now I'm not going to get all lovey-dovey or preachy on you, but there are a few things you should consider.

First, though, why a chapter on sex in a book called *Look Great Naturally*? Well, we all know that great sex (with the right partner) increases feelings of well-being and joy, gives us increased energy levels, reduces stress, makes us feel confident by boosting our self-esteem and makes us feel sexy – which results in more sex! Studies also show that people who have a regular satisfactory sex life live longer. It's thought that orgasm literally increases the white blood cell count, so helps to boost our immune system and helps us to fight off infection and disease.

You will have seen girlfriends who have a great sex life: their skin seems to glow and they have a sparkle in the eyes. If you're not lucky enough to be at it like a rabbit right now, though, or your desires or need for sex don't seem to match your partner's, then be comforted: you are not alone. Very few women are completely happy with their sex lives, and in some cases this comes down to not being very happy with their looks. A negative body image can result in lower self-confidence when it comes to sex, so it's worth remembering how gorgeous you already are, and putting your energy into feeling naturally beautiful and focusing on feeling sexy. So this chapter is about recapturing the tigress within, and spicing up your sex life, especially if you're in a long-term relationship and you've lost just a bit of that ardour.

SPICE IT UP

It sounds obvious, perhaps, but one of the ways to make an effort is just to remember how it felt when you first met. Remember when you were so loved up you couldn't keep your hands off each other? It's worth trying to put back some romance even if it's only in the form of leaving a little note in you partner's briefcase or a sexy message written in lipstick on the bathroom mirror. It's the little unexpected things that can make a difference. If you're brave enough to try some role play, dress up! You can have some great fun wearing some sexy kit, so that even if you both fall about laughing it can lead to intimacy. In fact, couples who share fun activities regularly are said to have more sex. It may be a bridge too far to study Tantric sex (I must confess I would impress myself if I managed an hour, let alone six!) but, flippancy aside, it's worth looking at a few of the basic Tantric principles – seeing sex as sacred and the main focus as being truly focused and concentrating on your partner. And where most of us (not just guys) often want to rush to the showdown, for lovers who practise Tantric sex the whole experience is important, not just the orgasm.

If you have kids, though, you'll know full well that you need to make time for sex. It's important, so schedule it into your diary. I know that sounds rather clinical, but if you're hoping that you'll both be feeling amorous when you crash into bed at midnight with your head full of what's needed for the next day's school run or how the hell you're going to get back from your meeting to make jelly for your child's party – then think again. It's far better to recognize that for a short time (well, realistically a few years while your little ones are very young), you may have to be a bit more creative. Agree to rendezvous early evening if the kids can go to a friend's or their grandparents, get a babysitter to come in on a weekend occasionally and make breakfast for the children while you have a romantic lie-in ... where there's a will there's always a way. Just one word of warning: put a lock on the bedroom door – you don't want questions about why mummy and daddy are playing gee-gees!

If it's all got a little more serious and sex really is off the agenda, be assured it's not an uncommon problem. Agony aunts say around two-thirds of the letters they receive regarding sex relate to one or other partner being unhappy with the amount of sex they have. Of course that will be different for everyone: you may feel hard done by if it's not every night, other girls are happy to have sex weekly or even monthly, but you will know if something doesn't feel right and there's a mismatch between your needs and desires and your partner's. In that instance, if trying these simple ideas doesn't work, I'd definitely recommend seeing a counsellor. Sex is no longer taboo and there's no stigma attached to seeking help.

Sex and relationship counsellor Rachel Foux offers her suggestions for spicing up your sex life:

'As modern women it's easy to become saturated with information about sex. There's a media avalanche of lovers' tips out there and it's no wonder that many powerful, dynamic and assertive women become apathetic or even embarrassed in the bedroom. Somehow this fountain of knowledge seems to strip away the pleasure from sex and replace it with a "to do" list. Sexual arousal is a natural body function, as is orgasm and, in recent times, research has demonstrated the many benefits to our health and well-being of having regular sex, such as an increase in immunity, stress-busting and burning calories.

'Left to our natural rhythm, the libido will ebb and flow through life and, just as we wouldn't want a sumptuous meal every night, it's unlikely that we'll always be hot for sex. One day we may crave something light and frivolous and on another occasion our tastes may be more inclined to luxury. Fortunately sex can be either gourmet cuisine or wholesome goodness, and as we are the chefs in our pleasure kitchen, it's our responsibility to find out what nourishes us the most, whether we're snacking alone or dining à deux.

'Sex shouldn't feel like a chore, which unfortunately can happen in long-term relationships; instead, let desire increase along with the knowledge that regular sex is anti-ageing. It literally makes you look and feel younger and more vibrant. There's no doubt that you'll be able to spot

a woman who's just had sex, as she's likely be oozing with self-confidence and sex appeal (and you're likely to hear a voice inside your head saying, "I want some of that").

'So can it really be that an orgasm a day keeps the wrinkles at bay? Can sex, lust and passion be more effective than luxury skin cream? Well, there's one sure way to find out and that's by indulging in a slow and sensuous massage, well at the very least in your fantasy. Sexual intimacy doesn't always have to end in intercourse, in fact it's sometimes more of a turn-on to build desire with good old-fashioned teasing, a blindfold and a feather tickler.

'Many couples are discovering more about what turns them on by playing sexy board games or daring to spice things up wearing just a diamanté-studded collar and cuffs. These days, adult toys, dare I say, are more desirable. Take a beautiful carved glass or wooden dildo, for example. These can double as pelvic floor toners and household ornaments, which have to be the ultimate gift of pleasure for women.'

— Rachel Foux www.sexandrelationshipcourses.com

CONTRACEPTION

Talking contraception just for a second, if you're a contraceptive pill girl, let me just point you in the direction of some further reading – see the section on planning a family (page 164). I'd suggest you also read up on contraceptive devices and hormone replacement therapy in the e-book *The Bitterest Pill* – www.centerjd.org/archives/studies/BitterestPill(f).pdf.

As times have changed, too, we have realized how essential it is to practise safe sex. If you choose to use condoms you can now buy Fairtrade ones made of natural rubber latex, though they can contain fragrances.

Try and ensure that your contraception doesn't interfere with the heat of the moment – if you use the contraceptive cap, for example, make sure it's inserted in good time rather than needing to rush off to the bathroom when it's all kicking off!

LUBRICANTS

A delicate subject, this, but we're all grown-ups! For some people lubricants can simply enhance pleasure or ensure lovemaking can last longer, but for others it's an absolute necessity, especially if you're experiencing vaginal dryness due to the menopause. Some cancers or even stress can make intercourse really painful, but you don't need to use the regular stuff in that very sensitive area, as there's now a fantastic alternative in the form of Yes! (great product name), a fantastic, certified organic, natural lubricant.

Traditional lubricants often contain synthetic chemicals. Yes! contains only healing plant extracts such as aloe vera (www.yesyesyes.org). There's a water-based and an oil-based formula. (It's not recommended to use oil-based lubricants with latex condoms as the oil can weaken the latex.)

You can also get Love Lube from Live Native: www.livenative.co.uk. It's a seductively aromatic 'all purpose' sex lubricant. It's non-toxic and free from any preservatives. In fact, the people who make it say it's edible, being a raw blend of essential oils. The coconut oil base in Love Lube contains three important fatty acids: lauric, caprylic and capric, which are all known to have antimicrobial, antifungal and antibacterial effects.

TOYS AND GADGETS

I know you're thinking 'Oh, please, don't start suggesting hand-knitted dildos!' Well no, but you do need to consider what the various gadgets are made of. Some are made from potentially toxic plastics and should be avoided. Even though these plastics (called phthalates) were banned by the EU from being used in children's toys, they are often still found in cheaper or 'gimmick' toys, and sometimes sex toys seem to fall into this category. Many manufacturers advise that you cover these sex toys in a condom when used internally. That's not gonna be great in the heat of the moment, so the good news is you can get natural sex toys from www.angelssecret.co.uk. Another supplier of a wide range of toys made from a variety of materials including safe plastics and stainless steel is www.babeland.co.uk. There's also the excellent Coco de Mer for all things sexy including lingerie and toys: www.coco-de-mer.com.

WORK THOSE MUSCLES!

A great way to encourage good pelvic floor muscles is to exercise them. Now, you'll remember if you've ever been pregnant that you were told to do your pelvic floor exercises several times daily, not just during pregnancy but for ever, but have you? Of course not! Seriously it is a good habit to get into every time you stop at traffic lights or every time your phone rings, let it trigger your memory to do a few ups and downs. If you're unsure see the Kegel exercises website www.kegel-exercises.com.

If you feel it's all rather too late for that and you could use a little help, or even if you're one of the many women who both before and after pregnancy find they suffer some leaking or incontinence, try the Pelvic Toner, a wonder device that is said not only to improve pelvic floor muscle function significantly, but also women find it greatly improves their sex lives!

You may be surprised to know that men, too, should do pelvic strengthening exercises, and Pelvic Toner sell a bit of apparatus especially for men – a much more robust stainless-steel affair – www.pelvictoner.co.uk.

Another rather unique product is the herbal vaginal stick. It's a vaginal 'stick' made from traditional herbs which is said to tighten the vagina while stimulating the body's own unique cleansing mechanism. I'll be honest, gals, I've got one looking pretty on my dressing table but haven't tried it yet. I'm just not sure if our wonderful girly bits aren't capable of cleansing themselves, and when it comes to tightening … Well, often lubrication is more of an issue. I'd love to know your thoughts, though, if you've tried it. They're available from www.secret-ceres.com, or you can get the Jamu herbal stick from www.herbalremedyshop.com.

Girlfriends' Natural Secrets . . . Top secret –

vaginal massage – yes, labia/vulva/pelvic self-massage using coconut oil. It's particularly nourishing before sleep. I make sure I do it every day. It helps to keep my energy moving. Interestingly it also seems to make my periods regular and pain-free. Doing the massage also reminds me to squeeze my pelvic muscles.

Girlfriends' Aspirations . . . Bareback horse
galloping in wind, rain and sunset ... on a black stallion ...
– **Rachel Foux, www.sexandrelationshipcoaching.com**

GIRLY THINGS

Well, granted, all of the above were girly things, too, but let's just talk sanitary protection for a moment.

I can keep this section pretty short. I just want to beg you, if you're using conventional sanitary products, to switch NOW. Regular tampons and sanitary pads are made from a bunch of potentially toxic ingredients that you do not need in that very sensitive area. If you usually use those applicator-style tampons then it's likely that in addition to being made from petroleum-based products they will also contain plasticizers, additives used to make the plastic more pliable, and this usually means phthalates which are proven to be hormone-disrupting.

But it's not just the applicator tampons that are a problem. Most feminine hygiene products use synthetic materials such as rayon, plastics such as polyethylene and polypropylene, chlorine bleaches (which release toxic dioxins), petroleum-derived superabsorbents, latex and skin irritants and chemicals such as fragrances, surfactants, lubricants and dyes.

The use of rayon and non-organic cotton fibres in regular tampons is thought to increase the risk of toxic shock syndrome. Tampons shed fibres to the extent that nurses conducting smear tests used to find they had to remove shed tampon fibres from around cervix in order to obtain a clear smear sample. There's obviously the hygiene problem of tampon fibres remaining in the vagina but also there's the possibility of vaginal infection from bacteria forming. When concerns were first raised over this, manufacturers tried placing a synthetic overwrap material around their tampons to prevent the inner absorbent core of fibres falling away during use and withdrawal, but the material used would be considered not ideal in that area either.

If you're going to use disposable feminine hygiene products, choose a 100 per cent organic chlorine-free brand such as Natracare (www.natracare.co.uk).

To convince you to choose organic tampons, try putting a regular tampon into a glass of water and you will see that within a short space of time, as the tampon expands, the fibres start to be shed. With 100 per cent organic cotton tampons, however, there's no shedding at all.

If you prefer sanitary pads again opt for the organic cotton unbleached ones with no plastics.

Washable Pads

If you can bear the washing (and it's really not that bad) then it's much cheaper and much kinder to landfill sites to opt for washable menstrual pads. Stop and remember for a second that our disposable society is still relatively new. Depending on your age, your mother and definitely your grandmother wouldn't have been using the 12,000 to 17,000 disposable tampons and pads that the average women gets through in her menstruating lifetime today. If you were to consider using a washable pad only at night-time, that's a start. You'll find a whole range and a great selection at www.moontimes.co.uk.

Menstrual Cup

Then there's the menstrual cup, which is possibly the most natural best kept secret.

Buy one now, and you won't spend another penny on your monthly cycle. They cost around £15 to £20 and work fantastically well. You insert the little latex 'cup' high into the vagina (and no, it's not tricky like a contraceptive cap is!). You can't feel it at all – well, not until it becomes quite full, then you know it needs to be changed. Then you simply empty it out into the loo, rinse under the tap and insert it again. If you're in the awkward situation of being in a public loo where you need to come out of the cubicle to use the sink, then you may need to improvise. Most of us carry a small bottle of water around with us now, so just use a tiny bit of that to rinse out the cup and then give it a proper clean the next time that's possible.

The wonderful added advantage of using a menstrual cup is that it seems to relieve menstrual cramps and, interestingly, it makes periods more regular and lighter. I can't prove this scientifically but it's happened to me and a number of close girlfriends. I do wonder if the absence of pain can be explained because regular tampons are so absorbent and, in some cases, so loaded with synthetic chemical toxins that they cause dehydration during blood loss, which results in pain and bloating.

In any case, a menstrual cup will revolutionalize your monthly cycle. You can buy the Mooncup from Boots or from www.mooncup.co.uk. Another brand is the Femme-cup: www.femmecup.com.

GETTING PREGNANT

I have to 'fess up here and now and say I certainly didn't 'plan' my family. I was a serious career girl who had absolutely no intention of having children. I didn't feel the slightest bit maternal and couldn't understand when I heard girlfriends talk of their biological clocks. How incredible, then, that I was lucky enough to fall pregnant by accident. That wasn't without its drama – I was told my first baby was an ovarian cyst; this was diagnosed after I'd been to the GP complaining of irregular bleeding, and it was only as I lay having an ultrasound scan to determine the size of said cyst that the radiographer announced calmly ... 'Here are a few small fibroids ... and this is your baby.' Of course there was still a chance of miscarriage, but in that instant my life changed for ever and I was suddenly very certain that I wanted this baby. I was fortunate enough to hang on to him, and then became pregnant with number two while I was breastfeeding number one! Don't let anyone tell you breastfeeding is effective contraception! Number three also came along unexpectedly, but number four was – sort of – planned (well, just left to chance).

As you can see, then, I'm not the best person to advise on family planning, but as with everything I have fairly strong views! I'd love to be able to wave a magic wand here and give you a simple, easy, natural, cheap form of contraception, but other than abstention I'm afraid this is one subject that's sent to try us. Perhaps it is for a reason. If contraception were too simple, perhaps we'd be even more promiscuous as a society and think less of the implications of having sex outside of long-term relationships. So I can't tell you which contraception to choose, I can only share my own experience. I think it's fair to say I've tried quite a few. I've used condoms, of course, the contraceptive cap (which simply flitted across the bathroom floor after what seemed like hours of fiddling), the female condom (which felt like a large plastic parachute), the honey cap (basically a regular cap kept in honey, which is said to be a spermicide but, apart from its stickiness, I'm told it's not very effective) and I've dabbled with the rhythm method, doing the whole deal with taking my temperature and keeping an ovulation chart (if this interests you, get a copy of *The Billings Method* – see www.billings-centre.ab.ca).

I only want to try and persuade you not to make the mistake I made of being on the contraceptive pill for many years. I'm convinced it's what led to me having an abnormal smear test, which turned out to be pre-cancerous cervical cells. I'm grateful for that incident because it gave me the wake-up call I needed, and led me to become interested in alternative health and well-being. I quickly realized what a fool I'd been to stay on a hormone-disrupting drug month in, month out for at least ten years when for many of them I wasn't even in a relationship let alone having regular sex! Even when I was in a long-term relationship, quite frankly we weren't at it like rabbits, well not after the first few months, anyway, so the whole idea of altering your natural menstrual cycle to the extent that you don't even have a proper natural period is like taking a sledgehammer to crack a nut.

I now really believe that it is a 'bitter pill' and I'd urge anyone to do huge amounts of research before they go that route. Try and be in touch with your own monthly cycle and its natural rhythms and don't mess with it. Go with the flow – literally.

When the time feels right for you to start a family, you'll be really glad you didn't mess up your system with the pill as you could need a year before you conceive after being on it. As I've already stressed, I'm perhaps not the best person to ask when is the 'right' time to start a family. I'm a big believer in letting fate take its course – clearly not to the tune of overpopulating the world with families of 11 children, but I do believe if you're with your soulmate, if you're stable and happy and you've agreed that you want children at some point in the future, then perhaps it's best to leave it to chance. Sometimes the intricate planning and plotting can lead to tension, which in turn means it takes much longer to fall pregnant.

I realize that with so many women desperate to fall pregnant it's not that helpful to simply say 'leave it to chance'. In this instance also it's easy for me to seem smug as clearly I fell pregnant without trying on four occasions. I do realize how blessed I am and I'm thankful every day. In truth I might never have planned to have a baby and then I would have missed out on the incredible experience. Don't get me wrong, I have several girlfriends who have chosen not to have children and they're very fulfilled and comfortable with their decision. Only you can know deep down what's right for you, and you should follow your heart. If you choose not to have any children, I'd just ask if you could offer your services occasionally and do some respite care for girlfriends like me with four, who need a break!

PREPARING FOR CONCEPTION

I've done a fair bit of research into natural ways of boosting fertility and preparing naturally for conception and pregnancy, and have co-authored an audio CD with a leading hypnotherapist. Why hypnosis? Well, I'm a firm believer that the power of the mind plays a huge role in whether or not you conceive naturally. Perhaps you already have one child but seem to be having difficulty producing a sibling. Sometimes the sympathy just isn't there; some health professionals take the attitude of 'Well, you've got one baby, don't be greedy,' but of course having one baby doesn't diminish the desire for another.

Of course when it comes to conceiving for the first time, none of us knows how we'll fare until we try. The irony, of course, is that many women spend years trying to avoid an accidental pregnancy, being diligent about contraception and panicking wildly if their menstrual period is one day late, but when they feel the time is right and *want* to become pregnant, frustratingly it doesn't happen straight away!

The good news is that there are lots of advantages to having a dedicated 'preconception care time' when you prepare your body for conception and prepare your mind for the enormous life-changing state that is pregnancy and then the birth of a healthy baby.

Nutritionally it's vital that you do all you can to provide the right environment for conception. Many of us find out we're pregnant only after we've spent weeks binge-drinking, and then agonize over any damage that might already have been done. The best advice, if you're lucky enough to conceive easily and without needing to think about it, is just be delighted and not worry at all. It's very unlikely that any harm will have come to your foetus.

On the other hand, if it takes a little longer then you have the luxury of time to plan, and then it makes absolute sense to be as healthy and prepared as possible both physically and emotionally. If you want lots of ideas for conceiving naturally, including nutritional advice, ideas for guided visualizations, reducing toxicity levels, timing of intercourse and where to get support and resources, then get hold of the CD *Creative Conception* (by me and Glenn Harrold). www.hypnosisaudio.com

PREGNANCY

Once you're pregnant, come visit my website! There's too much here to truncate into one small section, but I'm guessing you know my views. Pregnancy is not an illness, it's entirely natural and we should embrace it and focus on being in optimum health both before and after we conceive.

I'm a big believer in natural birth but I think as birth has become so medicalized in the UK the average girlfriend has to be really committed to a natural birth and do her own preparations. By that I don't mean simply attending a few breathing classes, I mean first off, addressing your nutrition. Most of us don't need to 'eat for two'. Reducing wheat, dairy and sugar in the diet, taking the right supplements, making sure you massage your perineum, using vaginal massage oil, doing prenatal yoga if possible and, if you can afford it, having a few sessions of reflexology and Bowen technique, all will help.

I'm a big fan of 'active birth' – being active and upright during the whole procedure – and, for me, having three babies born in water was fantastic. If you decide you want a natural birth and are committed to that, then the trick is either to opt for a home birth or to have the baby at a birthing centre/a midwifery-led birthing unit – there are more and more now, thankfully. If neither is possible, then try at least to ensure that you have adequate support so that your wishes will be carried out even if you personally are not in a coherent state!

Independent midwives are great, as are doulas (whose role is to support the mother, not to be there for medical reasons). A good doula is worth her weight in gold. She will be with you during the birth and post-natally, making you meals, doing the laundry, looking after other children – whatever is needed, allowing you to have that precious bonding time with your baby to establish breastfeeding and to rest and recuperate. www.doula.org.uk

I highly recommend that you steer clear of intervention, particularly when it's simply down to impatience because you've missed your due date. Babies come when they're 'cooked', and so long as checks show the baby is not in distress, my best advice is do not agree to be artificially induced, as this almost always leads to further intervention.

It goes without saying I have strong – some say controversial – views on everything from cutting the cord and eating your placenta (yep!) to washing the baby, breastfeeding, cloth nappies, carrying the baby in a sling and bed-sharing, but that's all for another book. For now I can point you in the direction of some wonderful further reading on natural conception, pregnancy and birth:

Gentle Birth Method by Gowri Motha
The Water Birth Book by Janet Balaskas
Birth and Beyond by Yehudi Gordon

Girlfriends' Natural Secrets . . . As soon as you open your eyes in the morning, a big genuine smile gets all the endorphins going. Then pull in your stomach muscles to the count of 20 and hold. You will never have to do stomach exercises again, ever.

– Fiona Robson, Imperfectly Natural administrator

Janey's Guide to Abundance

THINK YOURSELF GORGEOUS

Yes, it's possible! Most people are familiar with the term 'psychosomatic', the ability to produce bodily symptoms just by thinking. Well, the same goes for appearances, too. *How* we think has a huge effect on our external self. Scientific studies have shown a direct link between having a positive, optimistic outlook on life and having a healthy immune system. So thinking negative thoughts and going round with a 'glass-half-empty' attitude can actually depress the immune system. Low immunity not only makes you susceptible to illness, it creates that pallid dead-beat look that no amount of even the best organic make-up can mask.

Ever noticed how, when someone's newly in love, bursting with vitality and on top of the world, she becomes irresistible to all around her? Positive emotion seems to ooze from her every pore and infect others, making them feel good, too, and more likely to seek out her company. So beauty really does start from within, and can radiate from the thoughts we produce.

Beauty is, of course, hard to define, but it is so much more than the way we look, and there are many ways to be beautiful, too. We can be self-confident, giving, curious, passionate, vital, positive and loving. And these are all attributes we can foster in ourselves, without needing to go near the beauty counter or surgeon's knife.

So girlfriend, want to be beautiful? Of course we must look after our skin, hair, indeed our whole physical well-being, but we need to give our minds and our mental states the same treatment and kick-start ourselves into a healthier way of *thinking* as well.

I know it can be hard, though, to force ourselves to think positively if we really feel our glasses actually are half-empty! So how can we find practical ways to get back to a state of happiness without the need for years of counselling or therapy?

At the University of Hertfordshire, Professors Karen Pine and Ben Fletcher carried out some research that measured the extent to which people were open to 'new things' in life; how able they were to spot possibilities, behave flexibly and seize new opportunities. Karen says:

> *'We found that people who were more open and flexible had a BMI [body mass index] in the healthy range. That meant that, on the whole, people who thought in more flexible ways were likely to have healthier, more attractive bodies. Not only that, when overweight people were encouraged to do what they described as "something different" every day for a month, they lost weight, and those who'd suffered from anxiety or depression felt happier, too.*
>
> *'So the good news is, we can use this theory to enhance our outlook on life and to cultivate an outward appear-*

ance that's attractive. A good place to start is with the small everyday routines we have, because shifting these can open up unforeseen paths to greater change.'

The psychological technique Professors Pine and Fletcher have developed for this is called 'do something different' (DSD). Doing something new and different every day, however small, stops us living life on autopilot and nudges us out of our comfort zones so we are able to get more from life. Again, just like our diets and our skincare regimes, it's the small change/big difference approach. For example, have a day when you speak to someone you'd normally ignore, a day when you swap your coffee breaks for juice or exercise breaks, a 'gratitude' day, 'random act of kindness' day or even a 'no-moan' day.

'When people make small disruptions to their everyday behaviours, it steers life down a different track, to one that's healthier and happier. Journal-keeping itself is also a great way to consciously create the thoughts and behaviours we need to keep ourselves positive. The DSD technique really works when we want to bring out the best in someone else. We can't force others to change but we can behave differently towards them and, hey presto, they react differently back.'

In essence, Professors Pine and Fletcher's message is that if you want to get something different, you yourself have to *do* something different. Remember that not all physically good-looking people are happy, but happy people are always attractive! So the more we can cultivate a healthy, positive mind and a contagious, vigorous passion for life, the more beautiful we'll appear to those we come into contact with. And inner beauty is a lasting beauty, too. Whereas people get used to physical beauty after a while and its effect wears off, a mental beauty grows on others and lingers around for much longer – in the form of lasting friendships and loving relationships.

Girlfriends' Aspirations . . . My aspiration is to chase a tornado in America. Mad, I know, but something I've always fancied doing.

> **– Marie Barnes, co-ordinator of Breast Friends,**
> **a support group for young women with cancer**

MATERIAL GIRL ...?

If you believe that having all your material desires (or at least a good number of them) will make you happy, think again. When it comes to happiness, 'Give and ye shall receive' is the verse that rings true. If you're a retail therapy-style girl-friend, you may think that a good spending spree will lift you from the doldrums – but actually, why not try a 'giving' spree and see which makes you feel better?

A great way to happiness and gratitude, actually, is to offer some random act of kindness. Give away something you don't need any more. If you're the cake-making type, cut it in half and pop it round to the neighbours. Phone someone up and offer a free babysitting session (Lord, how I would have loved to have been on the receiving end of one of those!).

I once heard a wonderful story of a woman who, just after the Second World War, lost the jewel from her beloved wedding ring. She went to a Hatton Garden jeweller and asked him to put a piece of blue glass in there, as she couldn't afford a jewel but still wanted to wear the ring, for sentimental reasons. Years later when her adult son was helping clear out her belongings, he found the ring, saw it needed repairing and brought it to a silversmith, who pointed out that the stone was in fact a valuable sapphire! She may never have found out, but that jeweller obviously understood the power of a random act of kindness. Simply smiling at someone costs nothing, but it could change their state of mind, and have the amazing effect of making you significantly happier yourself. Making someone else's day, even in a very small way, can work wonders for our own morale.

LOVE YOUR WORK

If you don't yet have the job of your dreams, change your perspective and try to do your job with 'love'. We can't always have the perfect job, but we can still love our work. It took me years to lose the 'Thank God it's Friday' attitude, but most of us spend 75 per cent of our time at work so it makes sense to find ways to enjoy the moment rather than spending all of our lives wishing we were somewhere else. Check out the excellent little book *Fish!: A Remarkable Way to Boost Morale and Improve Results* by Stephen C Lundin, Harry Paul and John Christensen. It's a simple story of the Pike Place fishmongers in Seattle, a wildly successful business due to its fun atmosphere and excellent customer service. It's a tale full of simple but ingenious lessons learned from a place where the work could be construed as arduous and dull but has been transformed into a haven of joy and success.

Other favourite books to help you think positively and feel fulfilled include:

- *Feel the Fear and Do It Anyway* by Susan Jeffers
- *The No Diet Diet: Do Something Different* by Ben Fletcher and Karen Pine

- *The Seven Spiritual Laws of Success* by Deepak Chopra
- *Awaken the Giant Within* by Anthony Robbins
- *Stepping into the Magic* by Gill Edwards

Girlfriends' Natural Secrets . . . Be positive.

Personally I find that feeling good on the inside makes me look sparkling and great on the outside. I am fairly disciplined (most of the time) at keeping my inner thought processes upbeat and positive and to be mindful of when they might be taking a downward turn! Often people comment on how good I look when I am most in this practice! Bright, happy thinking IS the way forwards.

Girlfriends' Aspirations . . . It's a fairly big one:

that everybody has time and space in their lives to realize, without question or doubt, how truly magnificent and amazing they REALLY are. That the veils of separation and illusion fall away effortlessly and with grace and ease so that each remembers what lies within their hearts and has courage and strength to follow its call. When this happens, the world will be a magical space indeed. Just imagine people feeling connected to their inner riches and sharing their unique gifts with all those they are in touch with. We have the power to transform ourselves and our planet. My dream is that we each remember and make those changes NOW! It's already happening and it's so exciting!

– Priya Mahtani www.bluelotusliving.com

ABUNDANCE AND MANIFESTING

You know about cosmic ordering, I feel sure; you've probably also seen the documentary *The Secret* and been told many times that affirmations are the new rock 'n' roll, but does any of it work for you? Often we make the mistake of believing that all it takes is positive thinking, but it's just so damned hard to keep it up, especially when we're in the midst of economic downturn or personal stresses and strains.

For years I tried writing positive statements on cards and keeping them in my bag, my car and pinned to my bathroom mirror – but when I was feeling down they simply reminded me of my own inadequacy and imperfections. I do aspire to be a 'Pollyanna' type and simply see the best in everything and everyone, but I guess I'm really too realistic. When the chips are down they really are down, and it's yet another stressor trying to tell myself I look OK and that all is well, when clearly there's a huge zit on the end of my nose and I've just had the mother of all rows with a loved one.

Let's face it, if positive thinking and determination really worked, everyone would be feeling confident and strong; yet people who are gritting their teeth with determination to achieve something can often set themselves up to fail. Smokers who are finally trying to crack the habit often chart the days: 'It's four days and three and half hours since I had my last cigarette' they proudly announce. But why focus on what's left behind? Thinking about it all the time is setting yourself up to fail – instead, just celebrate the freedom!

I believe it's about changing your perspective. Without doubt the way you think is important, but I prefer to call it 'manifesting' or 'gratitude thinking'. If you search for the good in everything, you'll find the 'every cloud has a silver lining' adage to be absolutely true. When it comes to getting what you want in any area of life, you need first to identify in detail what you want and literally dwell on it. In his excellent book, *The Science of Success – The Secret to Getting What You Want*, Wallace D Wattles says:

> *'The moment you permit your mind to dwell with dis-satisfaction upon things as they are, you begin to lose ground. You fix attention upon the common, the ordinary, the poor and the squalid and mean and your mind takes the form of these things.'*

We all know that by trying to push negative thoughts from our minds in our quest to think positively, they usually come back to bite us. If I ask you not to think of a white elephant, clearly one will be lurking around in the back of your mind for a good while! EFT (Emotional Freedom Technique) can claim incredible results in re-training our subconscious minds. www.emofree.com

You must also set goals to aspire to. Write down exactly what you want, your hopes, your dreams, your goals, and review them often. Be sure to make them realistic – and then go after making them real. I do believe that if you set clear goals you usually fall just short of achieving them, but obviously if you set none – well, there's nothing to achieve or, indeed, praise yourself for.

The Vision Thing

I suggest getting a vision board. Any noticeboard or even a piece of paper will do. Just write on it six or seven things you want – it's OK to dream, but set it in reality. If you want to be a famous fashion designer, for example, realistically this is unlikely to come true if you have no ideas about fashion or textiles!

It's important to be specific: Don't write 'I'd like a new car,' describe it in full. What colour is it? What make? What's the registration?! Have fun with the process. If it's a partner you're after, beware of simply saying, 'I'd like a tall, dark and handsome man.' Describe his character, his profession, his interests. The chances are you will meet someone with a few of these characteristics if this is where you put your intention. In *Imperfectly Natural Woman* I talk of my friend who wrote her 'partner wish list' in great detail: where the guy should live, his looks, his character, even his financial situation. When two separate friends introduced her to the same man this was exactly him to the letter, all the criteria she'd listed were there before her in this man, who became her husband. There was only one minor thing she had forgotten to specify – he was bald. Of course, she was smart enough to know it didn't matter!

What Do I Want?

If you're unsure of exactly what it is you do want (and that's a surprisingly common situation to be in), a good exercise is just to cut out pictures and images that appeal to you from magazines, and maybe include snaps of yourself where you look particularly happy. Place them all around a vision board or poster and just look at it daily. See if the images lead you towards a certain dream or goal.

I'll bet you can think of an occasion when you really had your mind set on something, there may have seemed no way of achieving it but suddenly you meet someone who can help bring about the very thing you're after. I believe it's the energy you send out that helps to deliver to you what you need. When preparing to move house recently, I felt overwhelmed by the magnitude of the operation. We were moving from a hugely cluttered property into a much smaller one, without much time. We had a crossover period of about a week and our quote for a house clearance was hideous. While attending a parents' meeting at my kids' school, I started chatting to a woman new to the area. She and her family had just arrived from France and had literally no belongings with them. She asked if I had a chest of drawers to sell! I went one better than that and offered her a houseful of furniture for free. In return we borrowed her transit van for a week to ferry lots of things we didn't want squashed in the removal van. A classic case of the 'universe' providing us with what we needed.

The Wheel of Life

When I first tried to write my wish list, the words of the great Barbra Streisand song came to mind: 'I Want Everything.' My dreams wouldn't fit on one page. I now think that's OK – it's fine to have lots of dreams – but life should be a balance, so try and put things into appropriate categories.

You could take the 'wheel of life' approach. Simply sketch a large wheel, choose a number of spokes to represent important categories for you (career, relationships, finances, leisure, health are a few suggestions) and then write your dreams for each area. Keep to a maximum of six or seven dreams per category at first – it's a number we find easy to scan (more than seven and our focus can be lost), then work with each category in turn and draft an action list and a time-frame for each goal. If you get this bit right you'll be incorporating a useful time-management schedule into your visions and dreams, which all works towards achieving the outcome you want.

I did this wheel of life approach many years ago when I was out of work, in the wrong relationship and ridiculously ambitious. In the Career section I'd written 'I am presenting my own radio show on national radio.' (Of course I meant Radio 1 but didn't specify that.) It was a pretty cocky statement considering I had merely completed one short radio training course and was presenting a specialist gospel music show on a local radio station. I could never have guessed that a year or so later Richard Branson would launch Virgin Radio, and I would indeed have my own show on national radio for the next six years.

Mind Mapping

If you're quite a visual person you may find it helps to use mind maps rather than simply writing lists in a linear form. For inspiration, look at any of the work of Tony Buzan – *The Ultimate Book of Mind Maps* shows how you can add colour and illustrations to spice up your mind maps so that they look vibrant and help you to think laterally and creatively.

MANIFESTING YOUR DESIRES

Once you have your goals, create an action list of what you're going to do to set about achieving those goals.

Own It

If you've read anything on manifesting your desires, you'll know that the usual advice is to 'own' your dream, to act 'as if' it's already happening. In other words, instead of expressing your goal as 'I hope to be considered for an excellent position in a leading advertising agency,' act as if it's already happening, e.g. 'I am loving my position as senior executive with Saatchi.' Of course in some instances you may just feel too removed from that kind of 'success statement' at this point in time. If you're weighing in at 22 stone it may feel just plain daft and unrealistic to write, 'I am a size 12,' so a great tip is to 'own the journey', too: acknowledge your specific desire but admit that you aren't there yet.

Keep It Positive

Instead of saying, 'When I can stop eating too much I will be ...' A better, more believable statement for your subconscious and conscious mind would be 'I am now in the process of committing to the right diet and exercise programme to be at my ideal weight by ... [date].' In this case your action plan might be to join a gym, find a friend to jog with, and go and buy the healthiest fruit and veg you can find!

COSMIC ORDERING

If you haven't already done it, try cosmic ordering today. I had the great pleasure of interviewing Barbel Mohr, author of the original book on cosmic ordering, and she's an inspirational character. The whole idea of simply placing an order with the universe and getting everything you ask for seems just too good to be true, but what do you have to lose? She does point out, though, that our intentions and 'orders' need to be for the 'greater good', so there's no point wishing a rival company goes under so your own fledgling business is a success. There needs to be a good flow of energy!

- *Cosmic Ordering for Beginners* by Barbel Mohr

DIVINE INTERVENTION

You may find you want guidance and help to realize your dreams or reach your potential. There's a wealth of wonderful material available to you (check out www.hayhouse.co.uk), and you may also have heard of Angel Cards. Doreen Virtue, angel therapy practitioner and writer of several books on the subject, advocates these.

Angel Therapy (www.angeltherapy.com) is a non-denominational spiritual healing method that assumes that we all have guardian angels. It involves working with a person's guardian angels and archangels, to heal and harmonize their life.

Girlfriends of mine always keep a pack of Angel cards and simply pick one out at random when they feel they need guidance. It can be uncanny how the card seems to offer exactly the right words of wisdom.

- *Angel Therapy*
- *Angel Medicine*
- *Connecting with Your Angels* kit, all by Doreen Virtue

DOWSING

If you thought that pendulum dowsing is as old as the hills, you're right! Primitive cave drawings of figures dowsing with a twig have been dated as 8,000 years old. The website www.crystalgreen.co.uk tells us:

> *'The ancient Egyptians provide the first recorded evidence of using a pendulum, in a drawing dated at 4,000 years old, and they used them as a means of spiritual healing, the same as we do today ... The ability to dowse is mainly associated with finding water or in mining exploration; its use for that purpose became common during the Middle Ages and it is still used for that purpose today.'*

Many therapists use and teach dowsing to enable people to use their body's own responses to find the answers for practical questions. These answers are said to come from an 'inner knowing'.

You can buy simple dowsing pendulums on a chain for as little as £5. Choose one that appeals to you, or even use just a ring on a piece of string. I must confess I use mine in a rather 'doubting Thomas' way; I can't say I rely on it, but interestingly I can't seem to 'fool' it – I've tried asking all kinds of tricky questions and it sure does seem to know!

If this an area that interests you, get the book that explains the basics:

- *Elements of Pendulum Dowsing* by Tom Graves
- www.britishdowsers.org

YOU ARE POWERFUL!

Above all, don't underestimate your power for manifesting your desires and creating a life for yourself that is abundant and wealthy. By that, of course, I don't necessarily mean financially; you can be rich in many 'currencies' including friendship and love.

If you allow yourself to dream a little, and then realistically do all you can to achieve your goals, the chances are that your energy and intention will be focused and will result in the desired outcome. Just one word of caution: as the old saying goes, be careful what you wish for, because your wishes may well come true!

Girlfriends' Natural Secrets . . . *Have some me time! Whether it's half an hour in a coffee shop reading a magazine or an hour in a salon having a facial/massage/ whatever, FIND TIME for YOU!*

Honestly, once you get over the guilt you will realize just what those precious few moments can do for your renewed energy, refreshed mind, self-esteem (you ARE worth the effort!). And voilà! A more beautiful person!

– Tracey Hirons, administrator at Imperfectly Natural

Janey's Guide to Good Food

I've never been a 'lettuce leaf' kind of girl. I've always been able to rival the guys with the amount of grub I put away, and the bottom line is I love my food. After many years of faddy diets, calorie counting, and yo-yoing weight, though, I decided to look at the basics of nutrition and eating for optimum health. I discovered that the best way to eat healthily but still enjoy good food is by applying a set of very simple principles. This section is full of my top tips for how your food can be uncomplicated, healthy, fun, full of life-force and the source of the best fuel to do all the things you want to do – and look vibrant and gorgeous in the process! I'll list some of the excellent books on food and nutrition that have inspired me, and hopefully not only remind you of the basics but tell you how my whole outlook to food changed. I'll also share some of my favourite super-healthy (but quick and simple!) recipes.

WHAT'S WRONG WITH DIETING?

It's a sad fact that when it comes to food, women tend to think 'weight management' first of all. It's taken me years to change tack and realize that how food affects our *health* is actually all that matters. I believe if you eat a healthy diet – and I mean super-healthy – you will have masses of energy, look and feel fantastic and delay the ageing process, *and* your body weight will take care of itself.

I've never been obese, but for many years I was certainly heavier than I wanted to be, and often needed to seek out tops that were long enough to cover my wobbly bits! I've been back down to the weight I was as a 20-something for over two years now, and not a diet in sight.

I don't starve myself, nor am I 'superwoman' in the exercise department. So, first, what's wrong with nearly all diets and weight-loss programmes?

Well, the main problem is that they attempt to deal with *weight,* rather than *health.* A recent addition to the already overcrowded 'lose weight' market is the availability of over-the-counter slimming pills. It may not surprise you to know that this is clearly *not* the answer to obesity. The pills can cause side effects: one unpleasant one is unannounced 'anal leakage'. A friend of mine saw a poor guy in white kit who experienced that very unhappy accident. Not good! The manufacturers say that the pills only work in conjunction with a diet and exercise programme, and are essential for those who've tried 'everything', yet fruit and veg and exercise *will* work for everyone, so if the pill can't work independently, why not simply try the natural approach first?

Sadly, too, another thing the pills can't provide is *motivation.* I've heard a personal trainer to the stars say that the reason why celebs can seemingly lose weight effortlessly in time for a movie role is that they have excellent motivation – more fame and a massive pay cheque!

Even if you haven't resorted to slimming pills, I'm guessing if every single girlfriend reading this book had to stand up with their arms in the air for every time they'd tried fad diets in their lives, that would be one heck of a Mexican wave. I'm including the cabbage soup diets, the grapefruit before every meal, the F plan, you name it, we've all done it. Perhaps you're in the middle of one right now. If so, even though you've heard this mantra time and time again, I'm gonna tell you one more time: *diets do not work long-term.* Calorie counting is particularly insidious, because it's extremely restrictive and, simply because a food is low in calories, that doesn't make it healthy.

There's no point being skinny if you're unhealthy. Of course calories play their part. It's worth remembering that the earliest calorie-counting system wasn't devised by Weightwatchers or Lighter Life, but by the Government in the 1940s to establish wartime rationing! Interestingly, back then people were healthier, not only because they naturally consumed fewer calories (we all eat too much now) but because most of their calories came from locally sourced and unprocessed natural foods. Fruit and veg were home-grown and organic, the small amounts of meat and fish they were allocated were most likely organic because mass-production was not yet the norm, and the real 'baddies' – sugar and trans fats – were occasional treats only.

In the name of 'progress', by increasing choice and affordability, we've gone completely over the top and overburdened our systems to the extent where we think it's quite normal to eat sugary, fatty, processed foods almost constantly. The result? We're overfed yet undernourished.

The wrong foods – and that includes some 'low-fat' or low-calorie foods – will cause digestive problems, make you look older more quickly and weaken your immune system, not to mention decrease your energy levels and possibly give you mood swings. Over time you will find yourself with all manner of ailments that you'll put down to age, but I believe there's no need to be unhealthy as you get older. If you feed your body the right fuel, you can and will help yourself to fantastic health and vitality even into old age.

THE 80/20 PRINCIPLE

But you know all this already, don't you? If you're reading this book it's likely you've already ditched the kebabs, chips, Chinese takeaways and commercial pastries, apart from on certain occasions, of course. The 80/20 principle is good, and your body is able to digest and cope with anything in moderation, but when it comes to optimum health, research clearly shows that the healthiest diet is a raw plant-based one (that means fruit and veg) along with whole grains and small amounts of protein, for example in the form of fermented soy or tofu.

If a vegan diet is just not on the cards for you right now, don't worry, just take the balanced or 'Imperfectly Natural' approach and look more carefully at the foods you choose.

READ YOUR LABELS!

It's hard to find anything in our modern diet that hasn't suffered (suffered being the right word here!) some kind of processing, but a good place to start is the dreaded label. Manufacturers will do their best to make this difficult, with an abundance of technical names in exceedingly small print, but once you know what to look for, it gets easy.

The best advice is to aim for foods *without* a label – then you won't be going far wrong! The fact that a food has got packaging and a label often means it's been altered from its original state. OK, I realize that if you buy supermarket fresh fruit and veg (even organic ones) they will be packaged and labelled, but I'd argue that perhaps you should look at buying them loose from a local farmers' market instead. I've discovered that many of the local producers are pretty organic in their approach, but can't afford the excessively expensive certification process. Sealing fruit and veg in plastic doesn't help its lifespan, either; it's best to store it in brown paper bags.

We were designed to eat seasonally and the more local the food, the fewer miles it has had to travel. That's not merely a 'green' argument, it also means the food is likely to have retained its nutrients.

When labels are present, beware of their confusing messages. Avoid anything with colourings, preservatives, E-numbers (well, any chemical numbers!) and hydrogenated fats or trans fatty acid (animal fat).

Opt for accredited organic food where you can afford it. It's far more sustainable and will have greater benefits nutritionally. Try to avoid buying foods that have flown thousands of miles, even if they are organic.

Think Global – Act Local

Buying locally produced goods will make a massive difference to both the quality of your foods and to sustainability. Ask your local producers about the chemicals and additives they use.

To find your local farmers' market, go to www.farmersmarkets.net.

> Remember also country markets:
> www.country-markets.co.uk.
>
> Local farm shops are also an excellent source of
> local produce: www.bigbarn.co.uk.

LIVING FOODS

No, not that lobster still twitching as it sits on ice! Living foods are chlorophyll-rich and enzyme-rich raw plant foods. I'm talking really delicious and appetizing foods that haven't been cooked, microwaved, frozen or even steamed. They're in their original state and their live enzymes are still intact. So aim for sprouted seeds, fruit, vegetables, herbs, salad leaves and freshly extracted juices of all kinds (NOT from a carton – remember, anything in a carton has been cooked or processed, no matter how 'fresh' or '100 per cent' or 'organic' it claims to be).

Those who claim to eat a diet rich in living foods often also include wheatgrass, sprouted grain breads, delicious sweet treats such as raw chocolate cookies (which have been dehydrated rather than baked) and nutritious soups. In addition to a high proportion of raw fruits, vegetables, sprouted seeds and sprouted grains, most of us will want to add some whole grains. Remember, though, that the word 'whole' needs to be exactly that – where the whole grain is present rather than being refined and dyed.

Proteins in the form of sprouted grains will be more easily digestible than meat (more on sprouts later) and we also need plenty of good fats. Don't let anyone tell you that avocados are 'fattening'. They, along with nuts, seeds and perhaps oily fish (unless of course you are opting to be vegan or 100 per cent raw), are all healthy fats and are, literally, 'essential' fatty acids. I've got some fabulous raw recipes for you to try later. So let's look in a bit more detail at what you can and should eat for optimum health.

SPROUTS

One of my girlfriends paid for her student son to see a nutritionist after his acne was starting to really upset him. She was pleased to find he had really taken the nutritionist's advice on board and had ditched the sugary drinks and processed foods, started drinking lots of water, and was eating some good oils. What she couldn't comprehend was why their fridge was stocked to the brim with Brussels sprouts. When she asked him, her son said, 'The nutritionist said sprouts are packed full of nutrients, antioxidants, live enzymes, vitamins and minerals, so I bought lots.' Of course she'd meant sprouted seeds and beans, not the rather more humble (and 'windy') Brussels sprouts!

Sprouted seeds, beans and grains are literally power-packed superfoods. Amazingly for such a small food, they contain an incredible amount of nutrients. When the seeds germinate they come alive with nutrients and a vast array of vitamins and minerals. They provide a great source of protein, too.

Do you remember growing mustard and cress on blotting paper as a kid? Well, sprouting is even easier. All you need is a jam jar, seeds or beans, water and muslin or cheesecloth. In truth no one has muslin or cheesecloth to hand, and let's face it, elastic bands are hard to come by in the average girlfriend's kitchen, so my top tip is buy a sprouter starter kit: a big glass jar with a screw-on lid with perforations for the water to drain and a kind of ledge so it props up on a worktop to allow the sprouts to be rinsed not drowned. You can buy them in healthfood stores, direct from www.aconbury.co.uk or from Living Food of St Ives www.livingfood.co.uk.

If you're new to sprouting, start with mung beans or alfalfa, which will sprout in 4 to 6 days. Start by rinsing them well, placing them in the jar and covering with filtered water, then leaving them overnight in a cool dark place. To rinse the sprouts through, tilt the jar at a 45-degree angle (unless you're using the sprouter starter kit jar) and place in a sunny position. Rinse morning and night and, after a few days, they'll have little 'tails' of about 1 cm long. Store in an airtight container in the fridge and they're ready to eat in salads and sandwiches or to add to smoothies. When you're a bit more of a pro you might want to think about getting a set of sprouting trays, sprout bags or even progressing onto wheatgrass sprouting kits. A fantastic read is *Sprouts, the Miracle Food: The Complete Guide to Sprouting* by Steve Meyerowitz. He's known as The Sprout Man and is king of sprouting and the benefits of wheatgrass.

Libido Boosters

Forget the oysters! Most foods that are extremely good for you are great for improving your energy levels and, one would hope, your sex life! There are too many to list here but choose from:

- all kinds of berries
- avocados
- asparagus
- seaweed

- spirulina
- quinoa
- watercress
- and chocolate – yes, chocolate is an incredible superfood.
  Just make sure it's raw chocolate, and once you start using this miracle wonder you'll be in seventh heaven.

IN THE RAW

Shazzie, author of the excellent *Detox Your World*, describes
raw superfoods as 'ecstatic' foods. It's a good description of
how you'll feel if you eat a diet rich in these foods. Her book
Shazzie's Detox Delights is a favourite of mine for raw food
recipes.

Here she is with the raw foods lowdown:

*'When you ingest cooked food, your body acts as if it
has been poisoned. White blood cells are produced and
rush to your defence. This immune response is known as
leukocytosis. If you eat raw food, or at least 50 per cent
raw food in each meal, this doesn't happen.*

*'All forms of cooking change the structure of the cells
within the food. Your body has to try and do something
with these new and unrecognizable chemicals. When
your body has to deal with this chemical assault on a
daily basis, over weeks, months and years, it doesn't
have the time or energy to do normal housecleaning and
repair. It also has to find safe places to put the chemicals
that it doesn't have time to remove. This long-term stor-
age of toxins accounts for many of the diseases prevalent
in our society.'*

Most raw foodists are vegetarian or vegan, but some eat raw fish and meat. The benefits of a high-raw or all-raw diet include increased energy, needing less sleep, relief from chronic illnesses, weight loss (if you're overweight to start with) and a sense of well-being and happiness.

The misconception is that a raw diet means living on salads and fruit. This couldn't be further from the truth. There are now so many incredible superfoods and alternative ways of preparing raw food that it's easily as interesting and complex as a cooked meal – it's just a different method of preparation.

A great introduction to raw foods is to treat yourself to a meal at one of the amazing new restaurants that have started up in recent years. Saf in London's East End is one of my favourites: www.safrestaurant.co.uk. One visit there and I was hooked. It inspired me to go along to an introductory course in raw food preparation with raw food chef Russell James (www.therawchef.com). Boy, what a feast! We learned how to create, and then duly ate, the most scrumptious hors d'oeuvres, 'caramelized' onion roulade, 'roast' vegetable tart, along with various marinated and dehydrated vegetables including mushrooms with fresh pesto, yummy... followed by the best chocolate torte with ginger cream syrup I have ever tasted. Despite the conventional names the whole meal was 100 per cent vegan and raw.

But there's no need to go raw Cordon Bleu! Day to day, we need ideas for quick and easy meals. 'Raw foodies' tend to eat lots of fruits and veg (dried and fresh), sprouts, herbs and spices, seeds and nuts and their butters, grains and sea vegetables, and often add to their diet various supplements and oils as well as superfoods. For masses of ideas, pick up one of the excellent recipe books such as *The Raw Energy Bible* by Leslie Kenton. Get signed up to receive emails from Karen Knowler, an inspirational raw food coach: www.therawfoodcoach.com. See also *Raw for Life*: www.rawforlife.co.uk. There are also some inspirational videos and e-books courtesy of Victoria Leith, who calls herself 'the fresh and live mama' at www.littleguru.co.uk. See also the excellent book *Living Foods for Radiant Health* by Elaine Bruce.

GETTING STARTED
You can start just by making your salads interesting. The 'raw food fairies' – a couple of gals who will deliver the most delicious raw food to your door (www.rawfairies.com) recommend this great salad:

Raw Salad
Serves 2–3
- 10 radishes, thinly sliced
- 25 g dried arame (seaweed), soaked
- 1 avocado, cubed
- 6 sundried tomatoes, soaked and cut into thin strips
- 1 courgette, sliced into ribbons with a vegetable peeler
- 2 handfuls alfalfa sprouts
- 100 g salad leaves such as baby spinach

Dressing
- 1 large tomato
- 1 clove garlic
- ¼ cup water
- ¼ cup olive oil
- 2 tablespoons lemon juice

- 2 tablespoons fresh basil
- ½ teaspoon salt
- black pepper to taste

Mix all dressing ingredients in a blender. Toss all of the vegetables, seaweed, sprouts and leaves with the dressing.

Girlfriends' Natural Secrets . . . In the realm of beautiful skin, people may recommend a good cleanse, tone and moisturize routine with regular facials, but my secret ingredients are the juice of two cucumbers a day and a dessertspoon of MSM crystals in water a day. Our bodies love the silica and sulphur in these products and we get shiny hair, strong nails, clear and youthful skin as well as losing water retention.

Girlfriends' Aspirations . . . Apart from getting all world leaders to chant 'I'd like to teach the world to sing in perfect harmony' while holding hands, is for everyone to find their own personal stash of uber-happiness. It's within us all, and when we strip away our preconceptions, dogma, beliefs and outdated systems, the divine being in all of us really gets a chance to shine.

Bliss U

– Shazzie, author and Visionary in Paradise
www.shazzie.com

SUPERFOODS

You've heard this term a lot, I'm sure, and have perhaps searched for a definitive list. There isn't one! Different nutritionists and experts will label various foods as 'superfoods'. The simple truth is that superfood is any food that improves energy levels, boosts immunity and is high in nutrients.

David Wolfe, one of the leading experts on raw food, has written a guide to superfoods. He says:

'They comprise a specific set of edible, incredibly nutritious plants that cannot be entirely classified as foods or medicines, because they combine positive aspects of both and are an essential part of a balanced diet and allow us to get more nutrition with less eating. We know that most of the conventional foods and fast foods today are nothing but empty calories. Because the nutrients in conventional foods are commonly depleted through processing, we must turn to new possibilities for whole and balanced nutrition. Superfoods represent a uniquely promising piece of the nutrition puzzle, as they are great sources of clean protein, vitamins, minerals, enzymes, antioxidants, good fats and oils, essential fatty and amino acids, and other nutrients.'

David Wolfe's book *Superfoods* gives detailed information on nutritious, sustainable and delicious foods such as goji berries, cacao beans (raw chocolate), maca, spirulina, bee products, hemp seed and a host of others, along with recipes and suggestions for integrating these magical new foods into a transformative diet and lifestyle.

To buy superfoods and raw food ingredients go to:

- Gojiking www.gojiking.co.uk
- Detox Your World www.detoxyourworld.com
- The Fresh Network www.fresh-network.com

SIMPLE RAW FOOD RECIPES

If you fancy giving raw food a try, here are a few of my favourite, very simple recipes.

Sweet Potato Soup

Serves 2

1 sweet potato (peeled and chopped)

½ avocado

2 cups fresh carrot juice

pinch Himalayan salt

dash lemon juice

½ teaspoon mixed spices (nutmeg, ginger, cinnamon, or a ready-made Christmas spicy mix from www.steenbergs.co.uk)

Blend all the ingredients together until smooth. Either eat cold or warm up!

Mushroom Mini 'Pizza' Delight

Serves 2 (or 1 hungry raw foodie)

2 large Portobello mushrooms

tamari sauce

1 teaspoon tahini

2 small strips avocado

¼ cherry tomato

fresh herbs

Remove the mushroom stalks and marinade the mushrooms in the tamari for an hour or two. Add tahini, avocado, tomato and herbs. Yum!

Sweet Nutty Energy Ball

Serves 1

½ cup pine-nuts

½ cup dates

½ cup filtered water

½ teaspoon nutmeg

Blend ingredients together in a high-speed blender and then form into a ball or flatten into a kind of 'cake' – either way it tastes great.

Raw Chocolate Mousse

Serves 2 – 3

You won't believe this, but when I served this to my guests none of them knew it contained avocado!

2 ripe organic avocados (peeled, stoned and sliced)

½ cup sweetener (agave nectar or Sweet Freedom)

½ tablespoon organic vanilla extract

½ cup raw cocoa powder

Blend or process all the ingredients until the mixture is smooth You can instantly serve the mousse in individual ramekin dishes with fresh raspberries on top, but it's best if left to cool in the fridge for at least an hour. You can also add cashew nuts or ginger cream – see my website for recipes.

WILD FOODS

Nature can and will provide us with much of what we need, and in recent years foraging for food has become popular again. In some areas you'll find foraging walks where you go off with an expert, collect some wild goodies and then go back to a kitchen to create a culinary delight. It's a great way to meet and network with lots of other like-minded wild foodies! Even simpler is just to make the most of fruits and berries in season. See www.wildmanwildfood.co.uk.

Sea veg are incredibly good for you; if you can't forage your own, go to www.justseaweed.com.

JUICING – MY HOLY GRAIL!

I lost over a stone in weight in just under a year and am now the same dress size as I was in my twenties – what's my secret? Well, it was all kickstarted by juicing.

When I wrote my first book I suggested a few great tips for juicing, but in truth my juicer rarely came out of the cupboard and always seemed too much of a hassle to clean. My first experience of a juice detox retreat, though, completely changed my life. I learned about the whole psychology of addiction and the food trap. Even many of the recommended diets included eating processed foods. Most importantly, I learned that drinking freshly extracted juice is fantastic for getting nutrients straight to the body's cells. It's also a very healthy way to lose weight and gain energy. I lost about eight pounds in the first week and then kept up the momentum and lost a further stone and half over the next year, no dieting whatsoever, simply drinking juice daily and being aware of the 80/20 principle. By eating high water-content live foods around 80 per cent of the time, that still left 20 per cent for when I simply had to have chunky chips or a chocolate croissant!

Girlfriends' Natural Secrets . . . Hydrate your skin by 'eating water' as well as drinking it – by that I mean make sure your diet includes lots of fresh raw fruit and vegetables.

Girlfriends' Aspirations . . . I'd love to open a really sophisticated, sexy raw food café to show off how creative and vibrant healthy food can be.

– Christina Agnew, co-founder of Raw Fairies
www.rawfairies.com

Those suspicious of the health benefits of juicing reckon it's a problem extracting only the juice and thereby not eating the fibre, but the nutrients are in the juice. Fibre is, of course, necessary, but we do of course get fibre in other things we eat. One of the greatest exponents of juicing, Jay Kordich, reckons that fibre can't penetrate through the intestinal wall, so if you eat a raw carrot, for example, your mouth acts like the blender, the stomach is the juice extractor. Of course we need to eat solid food, too, but for many of us eating copious amounts of certain vegetables can be quite taxing, so to get the good stuff straight to where it's needed, juicing is the quickest way and puts the least burden on the system.

Girlfriends' Natural Secrets . . . A good blender and a dehydrator (see page 222) are the most essential items I have ever bought. They eliminate the need to buy any processed/packaged food. The kids love the homemade dried fruit, and I can make wholesome meals in a few moments.

Girlfriends' Aspirations . . . I would like to see all the small companies join together and overtake the multinationals so we again have small, interesting and healthy brands back on all our shop shelves in abundance. I would like to see chocolate counters containing only raw chocolate!

– Rajasana Otiende www.lifescapemag.com

Jason Vale, one of the leading exponents in promoting the benefits of juicing, has set up the first Juice Therapy course accredited by the Complementary Medical Association. See www.juicemaster.com for details and to find a therapist near you

Many years ago, Dr Max Gerson of the Gerson Institute became noted for curing cancer with a detox programme using juices and raw foods. See the book *The Gerson Therapy: The Amazing Juicing Programme for Cancer and Other Illnesses* co-written by Max Gerson's daughter Charlotte Gerson, who continues his work.

Buying a Juicer

There's a wide range to choose from, but the best one for you is the one you'll use every day. Masticating juicers such as the Champion, the Greenstar or the 'Norwalk' yield more juice and retain more of the nutritional value. Centrifugal juicers are quicker and simpler, with a wide funnel that takes fruit whole. They're also easy to clean.

Technique

Lay out all the fruit and veg you'll need; chop or peel anything that requires it. Most of the nutrients are in the skin or just below, so with most fruit and veg leave the peel on; the only exceptions are oranges, avocados and bananas. Make sure you have some ice on hand, too. The really important bit is to clean out the machine straight away so that the pulp doesn't get welded on; it's miserable to come back to a machine full of slowly rotting veg later on. Pop a biodegradable bag into the pulp collection bit, and don't forget you can use some of the pulp immediately for a fresh live-enzyme face mask!

What to Make?

Initially you should probably start with simple juices – fresh apple juice is a world apart from the cloudy cooked stuff in cartons!

Next try 'lemon' ade – well, it's 'apple ade' really. Simply pop in 1 apple, 1 chunk of lemon and another apple. (The Pink Lady or Gala apples work well.) Juice the lot and serve over ice, it will be a huge hit with the kids!

Apple, carrot and ginger is another simple favourite. Simply 'sandwich' a couple of chunks of carrot with a slice of ginger between two apples, juice and serve over ice. You can add lemon to taste.

The classic favourite, of course, is fresh orange juice. Better to juice it than to squeeze, as that way you get the nutrients contained in the pith, too. Combine with carrot and ginger and you have a winning juice.

'Shrek Green' Smoothie
- 2 apples or 2 chunks of pineapple as a base
- chunk of broccoli stalk
- small handful spinach
- 2-inch piece cucumber
- ¾-inch bit of celery (fennel works well, too)

You can replace ingredients with whatever you have – a couple of Brussels sprouts, some courgette, green pepper, pretty much anything can be juiced (apart from onions and leeks) and every veg has different health-giving properties.

Once juiced, add to a blender with a handful of sprouted seeds, a chunk of avocado and any other additions you fancy, such as a tablespoon of Udo's Choice or flax oil, or you may want to add yoghurt and chuck in three or four ice cubes, too. Whizz it all up together and serve – it makes a fantastic healthy breakfast which will keep you going for a good few hours.

The Amazing Avocado

If you're not a fan of avocados, they're worth learning to like. Add avocado to your smoothie to make it a meal; you won't feel hungry as avocados are very satiating. Obviously blend them rather than juice. Contrary to popular opinion they are not fattening, they help to regulate the appetite so you don't crave fatty foods.

Mix and Match

You can of course try any ingredients. Beetroot works well; it's great for cleansing blood and regulating blood pressure. Try it with carrot and lemon (it turns everything a wonderful deep red). In the summer try watermelon; it's 98 per cent water but loaded with vitamins and minerals including zinc.

Remember to add parsley to smoothies when you can. It contains B_{12} and lots of other nutrients.

I could go on for ever, but it's another whole book! I'll finish with one top tip for a winter warming drink. This is fantastic if you feel a cold coming on.

Ginger Shot
- ½ large apple
- big chunk ginger

Juice together and serve in a shot glass to down in one. Whooah, that is hot! It's amazing for hayfever and colds.

For a more soothing late-night version:

- 2 apples
- chunk lemon
- chunk ginger

Juice together, then add half a cup of boiling water and a spoonful of honey.

Ginger and Garlic

Fresh ginger is an incredible anti-nausea remedy, and also fantastic for relieving inflammatory pain and for helping with blocked sinuses. Ginger doesn't need to be peeled if you're juicing it or using it in a smoothie, so give yourself a daily 'shot'.

Garlic is another amazing cold remedy, and also lowers blood cholesterol levels. Use it in any cooking and on salads and in soups. If you need a decongestant, add it to a juice or smoothie. To keep the juicer from retaining the strong aroma for ages, juice an apple with a clove inside.

Learn More

Grab one of the many juicing books around to get you started. Any of Jason Vale's are good, especially *7lbs in 7 Days Super Juice Diet*. Following a seven-day juice detox programme is extremely effective if you want to kick-start losing weight. There are also good juicing books by Leslie Kenton and Michael Van Straten, as well as the 'oldies':

- Dr Norman Walker, *Fresh Vegetable and Fruit Juices*
- Jay Kordich, *The Juiceman's Power of Juicing*

On the Move

For the really time-stretched, try juice bars instead of coffee bars. Make sure they're making fresh juices, though; some juice bars can be rather sneaky and sell carton juice mixed with frozen berries. Granted, it's healthier than a coffee, but it's not live and kicking. I ordered a beetroot, carrot and apple juice recently in a fresh juice bar and was horrified to see the girl pour apple juice from a carton into the jug. If that weren't bad enough, she then grabbed and opened – I kid you not – a pack of cooked beetroot sealed in plastic! Thank goodness for the carrots!

There are companies that deliver a dedicated juice detox programme to your door, which include all the juices and smoothies you need for a three- or five-day detox as well as vitamins and supplements, aloe vera and advice and support.

www.radiancecleanse.com

If you want to buy juices and smoothies from the supermarket, opt for organic and choose the ones that say 'not from concentrate'. Of course most are heat-treated so can't retain as many nutrients as freshly extracted ones, but for when you're out and about Innocent smoothies are excellent. My kids love the little pure fruit pouches from Ella's Kitchen. You can add a spoonful of 'superfood supplement powder' to your juice to avoid any nutritional deficiencies – try the Live Greens from www.xynergy.co.uk or the excellent chlorella from www.sunchlorella.co.uk. Also vegan capsules or powders from www.naturalgreens.co.uk.

You can also drink coconut water as a great alternative to juice. Vitacoco use a flash pasteurization process; check out www.vitacoco.com. There's also Dr Antonio Martin's coconut juice from www.fresh-network.com.

FOOD GROUPS:
GRAINS

An intolerance to wheat these days is so common, possibly because it's presented to us in such an altered state. White bread, pasta and rice have usually been refined and will be deficient in nutrients – as will you if you eat them regularly! Be wary, though, of buying 'brown' bread, which can be just white bread with added food colouring. Most supermarket breads will contain a long list of additives, so if you're a bread-head make your own. Get a breadmaker and you'll soon get to know what you like, and you'll know exactly what's in the bread you're eating. When I first bought mine I agonized over measurements; now I simply chuck in organic flour, a dash of olive oil or organic butter, a pinch of Himalayan salt, yeast, agave nectar to sweeten and filtered water. You don't need to use sugar or milk powder, and of course you can add linseeds, pumpkins seeds, hulled hemp seeds – anything to 'up' the omega 3 count.

If you're lucky enough to get to a farmers' market or have a store selling artisan breads nearby, then try ancient grains too such as spelt and kamut. Rye bread is also good, but make sure it's 100 per cent rye – many 'rye' breads contain wheat.

In recent years the UK has gone pasta mad. It's seen as a healthy option, and certainly if you sneak lots of veggie goodies into the sauce it's not bad, but be careful of the 'empty' calories. Regular white pasta can be a stodgy old carbohydrate and isn't nutritionally fantastic.

To replace white pasta, opt for wholemeal, or better still, try the excellent corn or millet pasta from Orgran (in most supermarkets and health shops). Instead of white rice, which, let's face it, is really rather like school dinner rice pudding anyway, opt for whole brown rice or try Quinoa. Pronounced 'keenwah', this fantastic superfood contains amino acids and is cooked and used like rice. Next time you're feeling adventurous in the health store check out buckwheat, barley and amaranth, too.

Without doubt sprouted grains are the best. You can buy excellent sprouted wheat breads – sure, they have a label, but the one I'm savouring as I type contains one ingredient: 100 per cent organic sprouted spelt. You can also buy varieties with added linseeds or sunflower seeds, and a fruit version containing dates. Scrumptious. Try Sunnyvale, sold in health shops.

DAIRY

We weren't really built to digest cow's milk easily, but worse than that, over the years with intensive farming all manner of antibiotics have been added to the liquid that actually flows from the cow. If you're going to drink it, choose organic – but better still switch to goat's milk.

If you have any symptoms after drinking dairy (some people notice bloating and find they get catarrh or a runny nose), try rice milk or nut milk. When buying rice milk, oat milk or quinoa milk, though, be careful because they often also contain sweeteners in the form of apple juice and sometimes a small amount of oil. Not terrible in the scheme of things, but why not make your own?

Making Nut Milk

1 cup almonds (this also works with pecans, cashews and macadamias and, indeed, seeds)

⅔ cup water

Ideally, soak the almonds for a few hours or overnight. It's not essential, but soaking does make the nuts and seeds more digestible.

Rinse the almonds, blend well with the water and strain through a sieve into a bowl, pressing the liquid through with a wooden spoon. Even easier is to use a nut bag placed around the jug.

You can sweeten with agave nectar and add a pinch of Himalayan salt to taste, or use as base for raw desserts, etc.

Remember, too, that although milk contains calcium our bodies don't process it well. We're much better off getting our calcium from broccoli.

Butter versus Margarine

There's no contest. If you want to spread something on your bread, opt for unsalted organic butter. Better still, try one of the amazing nut butters such as raw organic almond butter from Carley's Organic Foods. You can also make your own: all you need is raw organic nuts, some olive oil and a decent high-speed blender.

Yoghurt and Kefir

Yoghurt slightly breaks the rule here, as many people who can't tolerate cow's milk are fine with yoghurt, and live yoghurt is loaded with beneficial bacteria. Make sure you choose natural, unsweetened and preferably organic. Even better, if you can get hold of it, try a live culture. I've got a blob of kefir called Horace; the yoghurt he produces tastes a little like beer, but all is well if he's mixed with a dash of vanilla essence and agave syrup.

If you're a fan of those commercially-produced small bottles of probiotic drink, you should try kefir instead. Commercial sweetened drinks contain one or two probiotic bacteria, but with kefir made the traditional way, you get dozens of beneficial micro-organisms. For more information www.kefir.net.

The best way to have your own 'Horace' is to get a culture from another owner. I have persuaded Dr Enid Taylor and she has agreed to provide a kefir instruction sheet and a small amount of kefir for a reasonable charge to cover post, packing and time to feed the little kefir blobs! www.taymount.com.

EGGS

Eggs are the perfect protein food. Just ensure that they're free-range and organic, and be careful how you cook them.

There's nothing high cholesterol about an egg; it's what you concoct with butter, cream and salt that gives the potential problems and adds on the calories.

COFFEE AND TEA

One of my personal battles is with coffee. We have such a café culture now that having a coffee is synonymous with having fun and being part of the 'in crowd'. Decaf can be worse; in fact, the decaffeination process sometimes involves formaldehyde and uses solvents such as ethyl acetate.

If you're a coffee-lover, make it good organic coffee, and opt for Fairtrade. If you've seen the film *Black Gold* you'll never again buy coffee that isn't fairly traded. Try www.cafedirect.co.uk to find suppliers of Fairtrade coffee, and for decaffeinated coffees and teas check the process used. Clipper brand teas and coffees use a method approved by the Soil Association.

I tend to like lattes or cappas, and have been known to have two or three a day, usually when I'm stressed. How daft! A bright girl like me knows that caffeine increases stress levels. I see my frothy milky coffee as my 'treat'. A psychologist friend reckons it's because I wasn't breastfed long-term and am still searching for that 'milky boob' substitute'!

There are some decent coffee substitutes such as Chicory Barley cup, Teecino and Dandelion coffee, but nothing hits the spot for me like my 'superfood' coffee substitute or 'maca laca' as my kids call it. Try this and email me with the scale of your delight – if you love cappucinos this is a pretty damn fine (and healthy!) alternative.

'Macacino'

1 heaped teaspoon Maca root powder

1½ heaped teaspoons raw chocolate powder

½ cup boiling water

2 drops vanilla essence

dash agave syrup

Put the powders in a jug and add the boiling water. Add vanilla and agave syrup.

If you like strong 'espressos' this could do it for you as a shot, but if, like me, you prefer a milky drink, add half a cup of gently warmed nut milk (or you could use rice milk). Use a hand blender to froth it up and grate raw chocolate on top. Yum!

Teas

Ah, a cup of tea, we can't do without it, and fortunately the varieties on offer are endless. Remember that regular tea, Earl Grey and some green teas also contain caffeine, so drink sparingly, but it's fine to drink herbal teas. Again, opt for organic and Fairtrade. Nettle and chamomile are my favourites (from the aforementioned Clipper teas and www.steenbergs.co.uk). You can also get a wonderful tisane from www.inlight-online.co.uk.

Make your own infusions, too. One of the simplest is fresh mint tea: just pour boiling water over a handful of fresh mint leaves. After a couple of minutes, strain and serve in a nice tall glass mug. You can add a slice of lemon or lime, too.

CHOCOLATE GIRL

'He knows she's a chocolate girl, 'cos he thinks she melts when he touches her' goes the old song from Deacon Blue (if you're not an eighties girl, excuse my nostalgia!). It wouldn't sound quite the same if it was 'Poor quality confectionery girl' – but that's exactly what most commercially available chocolate is.

We've all heard that chocolate is good for us, and it most certainly is – in its raw form. The problem isn't the raw cacao, it's the added sweeteners, fillers, flavourings and preservatives that make what's normally available a calorie-laden and very unhealthy choice. Luckily, however, I have a fantastic alternative: go back to its natural source and get into raw chocolate.

If you want to use it for cooking, opt for Willies Black Gold. It's fantastic for grating onto desserts, in milky drinks and for hot chocolate (sweetened with agave). You can also buy the pure ingredients and a chocolate-making kit from The Chocolution, and experiment with your own recipes: www.mayanmagic.com and www.sweetsensations.uk.com.

You can get amazing raw chocolate 'bars', ice cream and truffles from www.boojabooja.com. For chocolate flavoured with chilli, coffee, manuka honey and nuts, try the excellent www.nibchoc.com. My favourite is the wondrous vanilla and rose flavoured 'chocolate pie'. You need only need a tiny amount to feel satisfied, so it's a real luxury. You can buy raw cacao powder, cacao butter and cacao nibs from www.gojiking.co.uk and www.fresh-network.com.

A great read is *Naked Chocolate* by David Wolfe and Shazzie – see www.naked-chocolate.com.

If raw doesn't do it for you, then opt for high percentage cacao chocolate (preferably organic). Divine and Green and Blacks are the market leaders, but there are lots of companies now specializing in great chocolate. You can also get goat's milk chocolate from www.billygoatstuff.co.uk.

MEAT

As I said in my first book *Imperfectly Natural Woman*, I gave up meat a long time ago, but I am not recommending that everyone does the same. This book is not going to be a rant against meat-eaters. My own kids eat some meat, though I am religious about knowing the source. We joke about needing to have had a personal relationship with the happy, organically-fed free-range chicken/cow.

The secret is to make sure your organic meat really is 'organic'. Talk to your local butcher or supplier and make sure they know exactly where and how the animals are reared. Opt for lean chicken, turkey and lamb, avoid too much red meat because of its saturated fat content and, if you can avoid it, don't buy it processed and packaged, as those items are usually loaded with additives and preservatives. A good quality organic bacon should look the same once you've fried it up with your eggs, not shrivel up to half the size whilst secreting an off-white ooze. I have a friendly local butcher and I ask him about the life of the organic chicken before I buy it from him for my kids. Trust me, I tried to raise them as vegetarians but number one son toddled off and nicked a chicken sandwich at a neighbour's tea table the second he could walk. The butcher always delights in showing me his organic certification and telling me the origins of his wares.

Eating large amounts of meat on a daily basis is not sustainable either for the planet or for your health. You'll be aware of Paul McCartney's 'Meat-free Monday' campaign, and Dr Rajendra Pachauri, the world's leading authority on climate change, says going meat-free even one day a week is the 'most attractive' way for individuals to reduce carbon emissions. A recent UN study found that the livestock industry is responsible for 18 per cent of man-made global greenhouse gas emissions, not least because of deforestation in the Amazon – cutting down trees to create land to raise cattle to cut down again to produce meat. Financially, healthwise and from an eco perspective, you benefit from eating less meat.

VEGETARIAN PROTEINS

If you are already vegetarian, just be careful not to be too smug! I have a couple of vegetarian girlfriends whose diets are quite unhealthy, absolutely laden with fats and sugars and dairy products. Make sure your aren't overdoing the cheese and fatty, heavily processed ready-made veggie foods. Aim for optimum health, not simply avoiding meat. To make sure you get your protein in other ways, beans (fancy name, legumes or pulses) are packed with the stuff and are complex carbohydrates to boot, with the added benefit of containing no fat. Lentils are particularly versatile and provide more protein than red meat. Buy your pulses and beans from a healthfood store where possible and make sure they're organic. Rinse them thoroughly before use and get used to using them in soups and casseroles as well as in bakes and salads.

Tofu and fermented soy are wonderful sources of protein and make a great alternative to meat.

FISH
Fish can have health benefits if you choose oily varieties such as wild salmon, trout, mackerel and sardines. These contain good quantities of omega 3 and omega 6 fatty acids, which are fantastic 'hormone regulators', great for skin and in preventing heart disease. Just don't overdo it: oily fish can contain unwanted pollutants, but these are only a problem if you overindulge. You could also eat fish such as marlin, cod, haddock, sea bream, etc., as these contain the same fatty acids (though to a much lesser extent). Also ensure that your choices are sustainable. It's widely known that Blue Fin tuna is endangered, but many other fish are being over-fished, too. Go to www.fishonline.org for more information.

Buy the most local fish you can source, try and find a good local fishmonger who really cares, and look for the Marine Stewardship Council's certificate www.msc.org.

SWEETEN UP
Avoid refined sugar as much as possible. It's not simply that it's fattening, it has zero nutritional value and in fact, over time, will compromise your immunity, hormonal balance and could be an underlying factor in many conditions including Candida and adrenal fatigue – that's before you even think about tooth decay.

Don't be fooled for one second, either, into thinking that artificial sweeteners are the answer. I was pretty horrified when I heard a leading UK doctor promoting a leading brand of artificial sweetener. I can't begin to catalogue here the possible effects on your health if you take this regularly.

Aspartame and saccharine (and also msg) can have an effect on neurotransmitters, affect serotonin levels and, as one part methel alcohol, could be considered poison – after its introduction onto the market in the US, incidences of illnesses such as fibromyalgia, chronic depression, seizures, even brain tumours increased massively. For most people the effects are not instant, they're subtle and insidious over many years.

Avoid 'diet' drinks and foods at all costs. Advertisements featuring our favourite pop stars make us think it's cool to drink diet drinks, but trust me, you'd be better off with the regular version if you must go there at all. Remember that Coca Cola contains 7 teaspoons of refined white sugar – that's way more even than the builders working on my house requested for their cups of tea! Be careful, too, that some bottles of lemonade, even though not labelled as 'diet', contain artificial sweeteners in place of sugar.

Drinks and foods that are artificially sweetened should be avoided at all costs.

Read *Hard to Swallow: The Truth about Food Additives* by Doris Sarjeant and Karen Evans. Try and get hold of a copy of *Sweet Misery*, a documentary by film-maker Cori Brackett. You'll never go near artificial sweeteners again!

For when you just need a 'sugar hit' – and trust me, we all do – sugar from natural sources such as fruit sugars, in moderation, is fine. So eat fresh seasonal fruits, grapes, berries, apples, pears, whatever you choose. And if you want to replace sugar in recipes, my favourites are Sweet Freedom, a product which uses pure fruit sugars and carob and is a great alternative for people with diabetes: www.sweetfreedom.co.uk. Agave syrup, which is easy to use, comes in squeezy bottles and kids love it: www.groovyfood.co.uk.

Organic maple syrup is also good, as is blackstrap molasses.

If you like your sugar to look like sugar so that you can add a spoonful to drinks and for baking, opt for Xylotil – Perfect Sweet. It's five times sweeter than normal sugar and available from healthfood shops and some supermarkets. Honey, or brown rice syrup are also good sweeteners.

A great treat is to pop some organic Medjool dates in the freezer and take one out when you feel the need for a sweet treat. It's a bit like a healthy version of handmade chocolates!

Manuka Honey

I've covered the benefits of manuka honey extensively in my other books, so for now I'll just say buy it if you can afford it! It comes from very happy bees in New Zealand and has incredible antibacterial properties. It's worth having a jar on hand for any emergencies – when applied topically to minor cuts and wounds it's very soothing and healing (it's called *apitherapy*). You'll notice that it's given a factor number – this is its activity rating. Opt for the highest factor you can afford: +10 is excellent for everyday use, + 22 is incredible to use therapeutically. See www.manukahoney.co.uk for more information.

SALT

Beware! We need sodium to function properly, but too much can lead to high blood pressure and perhaps heart disease and strokes. Even if you don't add salt to food or cooking, if you eat 'normal' foods there can be high levels of salt already in there. This caught me out when I bought a few pasta sauces for convenience. They were high-quality ones branded by a celebrity chef, but each jar contained 13 grams of salt!

Tinned soup, baked beans, stocks and gravies, sauces, cereals and cheeses all contain high levels of salt, as of course do bacon and sausages, smoked fish and (needless to say) crisps and salted nuts.

For cooking, add herbs and spices instead. A squeeze of lemon will bring out the flavours in soups and casseroles. You can also add organic tamari, soy sauce or miso – all of which are salty but only need to be added in tiny amounts.

Best of all is Himalayan salt. This is actually good for you. Before I got into eating a diet high in raw food, I used it to make my chips healthy! It looks pretty, too, being a gentle pinky-orange colour. You can get fine granulated or coarse rock salt and its benefits include the remineralization of the body with over 80 minerals and trace elements essential to health. It's also thought to help balance the body's pH levels, and can lead to significant positive changes in respiratory, circulatory and nervous system functions, among other benefits.

For more, see www.amazinghealth.co.uk. To buy it in handy salt shakers, see www.thesaltseller.co.uk.

WATER

It's become the new obsession, hasn't it, carrying around a bottle or flask of water as if there were a drought? My hubby thinks it's a ridiculous trend and flatly refuses to take water with him anywhere, but for most of us, if we're going to drink as much as we're told we should, then we need to drink 'on the go'.

As a nation we're now spending fortunes on expensive bottled water and adding to the plastic bottle mountain in the process. But even if we were to switch to glass bottles or those made from recyclable plastics or corn, what about the quality of the water, and is it really so much better for us than a glass of good old tap water?

There are some excellent bottled mineral waters, but there are also some that are mislabelled. They can contain some bacterial contamination and, of course, the methyl chlorides and phthalates that can leach into the water and become carcinogenic.

When we were kids it was straightforward: go to the tap, get water, end of story. Now we have a huge range of expensive filter units: alkalizing ones, ionizing ones, energizing coils, oxygenated bottled water, magnetizing pads that sit under the water. There's also Tachyon water, said to revitalize and synchronize the water (www.tachyon-energy-products.com).

So what do I drink? Well, due to my recent house move I am currently doing more research into all of this (enough for another whole book!), but so far I have retained my tried and trusted under-sink reverse osmosis filter, said to reduce contaminants by 98 per cent. I'm careful to test the water regularly and change the filters accordingly. I'm aware it's not the most 'eco' of solutions, though, so as I write this I have just invested in a water distiller. It's thought that a steam distillation system is one of the oldest types of purification. Roman soldiers were distilling water 2,000 years ago. It's used by hospitals, laboratories and clinics where the purest water is needed. Distilled water is effectively steam that has been condensed back into water. The distillation process destroys all bacteria and parasites, and all impurities like pesticides, chemicals and heavy metals are left behind as 'sludge' in the boiling chamber – visual evidence of what you have saved yourself from drinking. It leaves only pure H_2O, which is near-neutral pH and has a true alkalizing effect on the body.

I'm put off, in truth, by the cleaning. The gunk left behind in the boiler is quite shocking when you think you'd have been drinking all of that otherwise, but I'm assured that it's a case of merely descaling it periodically with vinegar or similar. I've bought the Waterwise 400, which distils 4 litres in around 3 hours into a glass jug and costs around £225 from www.wholistichealth.com.

Distilled water does, of course, remove all the 'good stuff' as well as the bad, but my theory is that we get all the minerals we need from our foods and I'd rather be in control of that.

The water we drink is so important it's really worth researching this one in detail for yourself. For more information see www.waterwise.com.

See www.water-for-health.co.uk for information on alkalized water.

If you can't afford an expensive unit, then opt for a simple jug filter.

Beware of drinking your water at very cold temperatures, though; it can be quite a shock to the system. It's far better to have water at room temperature.

There's an excellent book by Dr Norman Walker called *Water Can Undermine Your Health* available from www.wholisticresearch.com.

When I'm on the go I fill up my stainless steel water bottle – please check that yours isn't an aluminium-coated one, because there is always the possibility of it leaching into the water, which has been implicated in Alzheimer's disease. I like the Ecotanka, it comes in various sizes with interchangeable lids from www.evolutionlife.co.uk.

If it's not possible to fill up at home I buy Deeside bottled water, said to be 'health-giving water' responsible for the longevity of the royal family as it flows near their country estate in Balmoral. It tastes great but sadly, as yet, still comes in plastic bottles.

KITCHEN KIT

Your kitchen equipment may not seem to relate to how great you look and feel, but if you save time in the kitchen you'll have lots more left over to do the stuff you really love doing. I love the idea of being very old style and natural, but when it comes to kitchen kit there are a few super-duper modern gadgets that the savvy girlfriend needs. First, two that aren't essential but are great for raw food preparation:

Dehydrators

A dehydrator consists (usually) of about five mesh trays for drying foods slowly at low temperatures. It's fantastic for drying fruits, making your own vegetable crisps, etc., but it's expensive (around £200). Excalibur dehydrators are the industry leaders from www.wholisticresearch.com.

Spiralizers

If you want to eat a high percentage of raw foods, you might want to invest in a spiralizer, too. This funky little device will turn your courgettes, carrots *et al.* into lovely thin strips of 'pasta'.

There are also devices such as mandolins, which slice a certain way, yoghurt/ice-cream makers, automatic sprouters, etc. But if we're talking essentials:

YOUR MUST-HAVE KIT LIST

Juicer (see section on juicing)

Blender for making smoothies (you don't need a separate smoothie-maker, they're the same)

Food processor if you want to create interesting healthy cakes, biscuits, bars, etc.

For years I bought nasty, cheap food processors which would start to smoke after 1 minute of trying to grind up cashew nuts. Imagine my delight, then, when I came across a kitchen gadget which did away with the need to own a food processor, blender and indeed weighing scales, a grinder or breadmaker (and, if you really want to go for it, you could even dispense with your cooker). I know I'm in danger here of sounding overzealous about this machine; I can only reiterate I'm not on commission! For those of you who haven't come across it yet, you must check out the Thermomix TM31. It's a super-fast food blender and processor that also weighs, mills, purees, makes ice creams and sorbets, chops, minces and emulsifies, kneads bread and pizza dough, and even cooks, simmers and steams! The only thing it doesn't do is bake or roast. Best of all, it has one bowl with one blade, so there's none of that annoying replacing different blades business or stacks of washing up different bowls.

I've since perfected carrot cake, biscuits, all manner of raw treats, raw soups and my own granola. I no longer need to buy nut butters, nut milks, sorbets, yoghurt, pesto or indeed any sauces, jams or bread rolls, and I can do a batch of raw food preparation quickly and easily.

Now, they're mega-expensive (you knew I was going to say that), and to buy one you need to get a demonstrator to come to your house (it's worth it – they'll cook up all manner of tasty treats), but if you consider the cost of a decent blender and a decent food processor, then it may not seem that dear. The website also has details of how to become a 'consultant' and earn one that way (by selling it to others, like Tupperware).

To get back to the main thrust of this book, will it contribute to you looking and feeling great naturally? I think yes, as many a gal has a certain glow when she knows she can knock up a quick incredibly healthy meal, snacks on the go and a cake for the kids' school fete with a minimum of fuss or muss. You can also blend your own DIY skincare.

www.ukthermomix.com

Here are a couple of my favourite simplest recipes, made even simpler with a high-speed blender like the Thermomix. If you don't have one, just adapt for the equipment you have.

CADA

This excellent breakfast is recommended by internationally known nutritionist Cyndi O'Meara. Plenty of energy and protein to start your day right. Serves 2 to 4.

C: ⅓ fresh coconut – no need to peel off the thin brown skin

A: 1 organic apple, stem removed, cut in quarters (including peel, seeds and core)

D: 4 fresh dates, pips removed

A: 10 almonds with skins on

With all ingredients in the bowl, mince by Turbo pulsing a few times. Serve with your choice of fresh fruit, yoghurt or seeds, or eat it on its own.

Tip: For a more almondy flavour, add 5 apricot kernels before Turbo pulsing.

Variation: You can use other fruits instead of or as well as apples – try pears, kiwis, banana, etc.

www.changinghabits.com.au

If you can invest in only one item for your healthy kitchen, make it a juicer. You can find them second-hand. A hand blender will do for most smoothies, too. By the way, what you *don't* need (ever) is a microwave – so perhaps you could go on a swap site and do an exchange.

POTS AND PANS

Ditch the aluminium pans and, if possible, invest in some good quality stainless-steel or cast-iron saucepans. You'll know of Le Creuset, but there are a few other companies who make great cookware, too. For baking and roasting you cannot beat the amazing stoneware from Pampered Chef. You need no oil to cook with these stoneware plates or casserole-style dishes, you can use them to bake everything from cakes and cookies to fish and meat very evenly, and when you're done no washing-up liquid required; you simply scrape the surface clean with a plastic spatula: www.pamperedchef.com.

CONCLUSION

For more information on the relationship between nutrition and wellness try and watch the following documentary films – *Sweet Misery: A Poisoned World*, *Processed People* and *Food Matters*.

Janey's Guide to Alcohol

There will be many a girl who will have turned straight to this chapter. About four years ago it would have been the first port of call for me, desperate to see if other 'intelligent switched-on but boozy girlfriends' drank as much as me and yet still considered themselves healthy and couldn't bear the thought of being out of control.

The reality is alcohol is probably more damaging than many class A drugs, but most of us come to it at some point or other, and once you have the taste for it, it can be a rocky road to travel. Here is a naturopathic doctor's explanation of why alcohol affects us so badly:

'Alcohol is the toxin produced when yeasts have digested the sugar present in fruit and grains. The word "intoxication" literally means poisoning. Our livers have to work very hard to metabolize (detox) the toxic alcohol from our bodies. It therefore diverts the liver from its normal activities which is then allowing things like free radicals and other by-products of normal metabolism to

go unchecked. So whilst your liver is coping with alcohol and de-toxing you from that, it is not saving you from the damage of the free radicals and this can be accelerating the ageing process. Alcohol therefore speeds up the ageing process biochemically. It also makes you dehydrated which physically dries out the precious moisture from our skins, making the skin sag and wrinkle prematurely.

'These are the effects you can see on the outside, the internal effects are just as undesirable but obviously hidden. If you know somebody who has a severe alcohol problem, chances are their skin is finely wrinkled making them look much older than their years. Alcohol depresses normal functions and can cause depression (after the initial high). We seem to get high initially because we are seeking more and more stimulation from our environments to counteract the depression of activity within. It is paradoxical, we think it revs us up but it does the opposite.'

– Dr Enid Taylor, naturopath

Alcohol kills around 40,000 people a year in the UK, but it's also big business. It's seen as quite normal to drink regularly to excess, and there will always be glamorous adverts for alcohol, so that it can seem like the cool thing to do. We're led to believe that alcohol helps us to relax, but if that were the case, more alcohol would be offered to drunken guys fighting to help break up the row! We're sold the line, too, that alcohol in moderation is good for us, especially red wine because it's high in antioxidants. Er – hold on – it's the red grapes on their own that are incredibly good!

Rather than being 'under the influence' of alcohol, its manufacturers and the advertising industry, I prefer to make my own choices now.

EXCESS ALCOHOL IS AGEING!

Drinking too much causes lethargy, batters our liver and kidneys, makes us fat and a bit depressed, shrinks the brain, can lead to diabetes and heart disease, and causes impotence in men. It costs a fortune, often contains a hair-raising number of chemicals (I've never understood why ingredients aren't listed on wine) and means we can't drive home after a night out. It also leads to what I call the 'Oh, I may as well have it' factor. By that I mean that after a few drinks you make all kinds of poor food choices that you wouldn't otherwise make, usually because you're craving carbohydrates to mop up the damage! I'd consume far too much cheese or sugary, fatty foods; for many gals it's chips or kebabs.

We acquire the taste for alcohol; it's a learned habit – which is good news because it means it can be unlearned! Do you remember when you had your very first alcoholic drink? Did you swirl it around the glass and say 'Mmm … a good vintage?' Unlikely – I seem to remember spitting it out and vowing I would never touch the stuff again!

Do you consider yourself an alcoholic? Unless you're swigging meths at 10 a.m., probably not, but you'll be well aware of the Government guidelines for alcohol units. Basically for women it's 14 units a week. Now, a unit is one *small* glass of wine or one measure of spirit. That's a small glass, I repeat, not the whacking great glasses that we now love to quaff from. I remember when a glass of wine was exactly that, one glass and I felt slightly tiddly. It wasn't long, though, before that became a large glass, then two. For many years I became a bit of wine connoisseur (well, so I thought) and would buy all kinds of wines to drink at home. Most nights my partner and I shared a bottle of wine and occasionally, if he was out, I'd open a bottle for myself. Sometimes I'd have drunk two-thirds of it before I realized this was actually a bit sad.

It was quite commonplace for me to wake up feeling groggy – not hungover, exactly, I was able to function, but I often had a headache, diarrhoea (charming – sorry!) and felt slightly tearful and irritable. I don't think what I was doing was in any way unusual; in fact when I mention it to most of my girlfriends they intimated life was the same for them. Even when I had kids it carried on; while the first two were very young, like so many mothers with young children I felt absolutely frazzled and was watching the clock till it seemed an acceptable hour to have my first alcoholic drink. I used to joke with other mums about the expression ... 'Don't drink till the sun goes over the yard arm'... We used to say 6 p.m. was reasonable!

So you get the picture, and I'd guess it's not an uncommon one at all. As I started writing books about health and well-being, I started to feel anxious about my drinking but had no idea how to stop. I thought I had an addictive personality and perhaps I was a low-level alcoholic. I'd try giving up for a week or so but I felt miserable at being deprived, which in turn made me feel more stressed.

So what changed everything? A book.

It's funny, isn't it, how books, if you read the right one at the right time, can be life-changing? I picked up *Stop Drinking for Life – Easily* by Jason Vale and read it cover to cover in a day. It's a powerful book. Many people who read it do stop drinking for life, literally, and almost everyone changes their relationship with alcohol so that it no longer 'controls' them. I stopped drinking for around five months and didn't miss it one bit. Since that time I do drink wine again, but certainly not every day, and I never drink alcohol at home.

I can't overstate how it's changed me. I don't feel 'controlled' any more, I can now drive to parties or events if I want to without the fear of being stopped or needing to carefully monitor my intake of alcohol. I save a small fortune and my skin is better, I have more energy and have lost weight; I can also easily get up early without ever feeling groggy.

SOUNDS TOO SIMPLE?

The premise is that the physical addiction, like any other physical addiction, is temporary; it can be removed from the body in three or four days maximum. After the shaking and withdrawal symptoms have gone, the biggest barrier to success is not the physical craving – whether that be for an alcoholic drink or for a cigarette – it's the psychological one. Our brain is feeling deprived, telling us we could be having a better time, feeling more relaxed, more happy, telling us we're more sexy and more fun to be around when we've had a drink. The reverse is usually true – if you've ever been the only sober person at a party, you'll know how stupid drunk people act.

All it takes is changing that mindset. The majority of people who drink alcohol have no idea that they are in a trap. It's one of the subtlest traps ever devised and has fooled millions for generations. Gen up on all the information and then be clear about whether you want to drink or not. Without doubt your body does not 'need' a drink, it has no benefits whatsoever, so it's simply, do you choose to, or not? Jason Vale makes a very brave statement: 'There is no such thing as an alcoholic and there is no such disease as alcoholism!'

I can only urge you to read the book, which has been updated and is now called *Kick the Drink ... Easily!*

You could also go and seek out help. Hypnosis and NLP (neurolinguistic programming) have achieved great results with helping people to give up the booze.

WHAT TO DRINK INSTEAD?

Drinking alcohol is so closely linked to social occasions, and one of the difficulties of giving up is that you don't want to be the only party-pooper, turning up for a dinner party with your soft drink. Nor are lemonades and colas healthy or good substitutes. A fantastic alternative, though, is alcohol-free wine.

Now, if you're remembering back a few years to when you may have been offered a non-alcoholic wine, forget that experience. That stuff, along with most of the non-alcoholic beers, tasted like bad water! *De-alcoholized* wine tastes, well, like wine – it's just had the alcohol extracted. When I want to 'drink' with everyone else at a dinner party I crack open my fantastic bottle of pink bubbly. It looks gorgeous, in a proper bottle with a cork, and tastes – well, just like regular pink fizz, but without the alcohol – luxury without the headache!

I buy the Pearl Rosé Alcohol Free from www.lono.co.uk. They have a fantastic range of whites, reds and beers, too, as do www.thealcoholfreeshop.co.uk. If you have local bars or restaurants that you regularly frequent, get them to order in some of your favourite de-alcoholized wine. It's brilliant to be able to offer the 'drivers' of any party a more interesting option than the usual soft drink or orange juice.

THE RIGHT GLASS!

It may sound daft, but all the associations around alcohol are important, too. If you go out with a friend for dinner and they order wine, it will come in a nice large wine glass. Your sparkling water, on the other hand, will be served in a very plain tumbler. Somehow you feel drawn to the wine, but imagine if it were the other way round? Warm white wine in a tumbler or paper cup never did it for me even when I was a heavy drinker, so the answer is, ask for a nice glass! Treat yourself to a lovely wine glass with sparkling water, and a twist of lemon. Of course it's all psychological, but it makes us feel more sociable and grown-up!

MAKE IT ORGANIC

For when you do drink, choose good organic Fairtrade drinks. You may also want to opt for biodynamic wine. Organic wines are made from grapes cultivated without synthetic fungicides, herbicides or fertilizers. Also there are fewer sulphates, which usually means fewer headaches. You can also get good organic beer and ciders.

For a great range of organic wines and vegan, vegetarian and biodynamic wine, check out:

- www.vintageroots.co.uk
- www.vinceremos.co.uk
- www.organic-champagne.co.uk

PREVENTING THE DAMAGE, AND HANGOVER CURES

Water, water and drink more water. It's a good idea to drink water *before* alcohol, to slow down the absorption rate, and *alongside* alcohol as well. On the Continent alcoholic drinks are often automatically served with a glass of water – always remember, one glass of water for every alcoholic drink. And of course, drink copious amounts of water after drinking before you retire to bed. The ill effects of alcohol are mostly because your poor body is severely dehydrated. Taking the herbal remedy milk thistle when you are going to drink is a good idea and can help your liver regenerate more quickly. Keep some to hand for Christmas time or celebrations! (Obviously not drinking so much alcohol would be even better!)

Before you go to bed, also take 1,000 mg of vitamin C. See the chapter Staying Well for a refreshing hangover aromatherapy blend.

Girlfriends' Natural Secrets ... For more than

20 years I have drunk litres of water every day – at first it was to help me curb my appetite and help my skin.

I do feel that living as alkaline as possible really does help with natural beauty – I would never eat meat or dairy and I do feel that these 'food' products are ageing.

Looking into juicing and eating more raw foods is such an eye opener too – all of the raw foodie people I have met and seen pictures of look amazing with glowing skin too. You are what you eat!

Girlfriends' Aspirations ... My aspiration is simply

that my project VeggieVision TV grows and I can work on it full time.

– Karin Ridgers www.veggievision.tv

Janey's Guide to Looking After Your Home

This book is about looking great (and feeling great) naturally, so does it matter what our homes say about us? Well, yes – it all connects up. You may be renting a room in a shared house, have a houseboat on the canal or, indeed, be living in your dream home, but what matters is, does it feel like 'home'? There are so many simple touches anyone can make to even the most temporary space to make it her own. It is important that we come home every day and feel 'at home'; it helps us on the way to feeling stable and secure.

We all have absolute choice over the decor of our home. Now, if you're a student nurse in campus accommodation you may be shouting, 'I don't think so,' but I'm not talking about the wallpaper, the flooring or even the furnishings. I'm talking about the 'atmosphere', the first impression that can be created from – if necessary – the cheapest items, fabrics, antiques and artefacts. We've all been to houses or even mansions which look grand and opulent from the outside but, once inside, feel lonely and cold. We've also all been into extremely humble abodes where the feeling was one of warmth and welcome. It's largely to do, of course, with the energy of the inhabitants, but it's possible to provide a few visual representations of the positive energy, even if you're not particularly creative and have very little money to spend.

Furnishing and decorating your home is a wonderful way of expressing yourself, and it doesn't need to cost much money. Fortunately caring about the planet means you will want to eschew buying new wherever possible, so trawl junk shops, auctions and charity shops a-go-go, and pat yourself on the back whilst ticking the 'sustainability' box every time you happen upon the perfect old bookshelf for a tenner, or that great offcut of fabric that will look perfect draped over your 'vintage' couch.

'Reduce/reuse/recycle' is the mantra we've all heard, but when it comes to our homes it really does permeate everyday living. Once we start to ditch the disposables – everything from kitchen rolls, throwaway barbecues, disposable plates, batteries and cheap clothing through to sanitary protection – we start to think differently. By reusing our plastic bottles, refashioning something from a container, recycling – not just by putting our cartons in the direction of the 'cartons section' for the refuse collectors, but also by passing on unwanted gifts and creating an art statement or scarecrow from the boxes of old CDs (OK, he's a fairly futuristic looking scarecrow!) we can start to appreciate the fragility of our planet and also feel richer indeed. Salvaged and reclaimed materials look far more interesting and unique than an MDF item, and if you can frequent your local junk shops you could find some great sturdy furniture that you can sand down or give a coat of paint for a new lease of life.

If you want to commission a really unique piece of re-claimed furniture see www.my-kea.co.uk.

I'm not suggesting you have to be 'scruffy', just to real-ize that whether you are commissioning a new kitchen or a single item of furniture you can usually seek out sustainable choices that will look individual and stylish.

I've got a couple of wealthy girlfriends whose homes are im-maculate and have state-of-the-art kitchens and bathrooms, pristine new furniture, fitted units, designer sofas with the latest colour scheme on the cushions and throws, designer rugs and original or limited edition artwork. I also have friends who live in comparatively frugal surroundings, with sparse furnishings and, amongst the accessories, ornaments and crockery, abso-lutely nothing is matching. Can you guess where I feel most comfortable? In the humble cottage my friend has stuck fa-vourite photos from the last ten years of her life across one wall. It tells an amazing story, She also has a 'vision board' (see page 178), with all her hopes and aspirations represented in pictures or photographs. She's painted another wall bright yellow, cut up old charity-shop curtains to cover her cushions in gold chintz, and found some cute and intriguing wooden artefacts that sit proudly above her open fire, which she stokes by taking her dog for walks through the forest to gather wood, keeping fit in the process. The whole space feels vibrant and homely.

START SMALL

So where can we take back control? Well, unless you're lucky enough to be able to refurbish an eco-home with energy-saving appliances, solar panels, a wind turbine, grey water systems and sustainable materials throughout, then it's best to start small and save some cash in the process.

Financial solvency isn't the main issue here, though, it's passion for life and the desire to want to be healthy, happy and express something of who you are in your surroundings. Once you've sorted your recycled furnishings, look for reclaimed fabric remnants, too. Don't throw anything away; you can reuse everything. Old fabrics and cushions can be used to stuff a long piece of fabric for a draught excluder, curtains can be made into clothes or accessories (see the chapter on ethical fashion) and even old bits of carpet can be used to contribute to the compost heap.

If you're buying new, then again think sustainable when it comes to fabrics, not only in order to reduce your carbon footprint but to keep you well, too. For example, a plastic shower curtain gets horribly mouldy and mildewed, but if you opt for a hemp shower curtain it will be fantastically anti-bacterial and look great.

Hemp is a fabulously eco fabric and works great too for bedlinens and cushion covers:

— www.drapersorganiccotton.co.uk
— www.hempsolutions.co.uk
— www.finecottoncompany.com – for gorgeous organic cotton bedlinen
— www.serenitysilk.co.uk – 100 per cent silk-filled duvets and bedlinen
— www.thecurtainexchange.net – for high-quality new and recycled curtains at bargain prices

Girlfriends' Natural Secrets ... *If I'm feeling lethargic and/or down or if my skin has become very dry, I* up my intake of omega 3 (I have an underactive thyroid so my skin is prone to dryness).

Also I have naturally very curly hair and used to suffer frequently from 'bed hair' until I was given pure silk pillowcases. They have really made a difference! Also the feel of the silk on my face and the coolness of the fabric are luxurious. I would love to sleep wrapped in pure silk sheets every night!

– Jo Lunn, Bowen technique practitioner

CLEANING

How you clean and care for your home is very much connected with looking and feeling great. We know the average home is more polluted than a busy street corner, and while we can't do much about the traffic and airborne pollution, we can certainly make sustainable healthy choices in what we use to clean and refresh our personal space.

First we need to accept that synthetic chemicals, pesticides and pollutants are everywhere: in our furnishings, carpets, the paint on our walls, our cleaning and personal care products. Add to that the effects of 'electro-pollution' – the cumulative effects of our electrical items and wi-fi technology – and it's no wonder that so many of us are prone to headaches and low-level fatigue.

If you've read the skincare chapter you'll know I have suggested do-it-yourself recipes using what's already in the average kitchen cupboard. For cleaning it's no different, you can easily make your own concoctions, or if you choose to buy, then go for one of the more natural options.

What's Wrong with Conventional Detergents?

Just about everything! They're unsustainable, many are petrochemical based (and petrol is a non-renewable resource, harmful to the environment), they contaminate rivers and seas, many contain chemicals which are creating strong superbugs and an unbalanced ecosystem. They also contribute to ill health and, in the case of laundry products, can be a skin irritant and lead to allergies, too.

Let's get to the good news: there are a wealth of great plant-based alternatives for cleaning our homes and clothes.

Air Fresheners

Let's start with freshening the air. Studies have shown that women who work in the home have a 55 per cent increased risk of getting cancer. Research also shows that women suffer from headaches largely due to VOCs – (volatile organic compounds, which will also aggravate anyone with respiratory conditions such as asthma) and the artificial fragrances which can be hormone-disrupting. VOCs are found in a host of household products including paints, aerosol sprays, cleansers, disinfectants, air fresheners and dry-cleaned clothing!

We've forgotten the obvious one when it comes to air freshening – open the window! Most of us live in sealed units where we've triple-glazed, have the radiators on full and wonder why we can't shake off infections. Open the windows wide, especially when you clean the house! No one needs ever again to buy air freshener, neither an aerosol nor those scary plug-in ones. Simply get a plant sprayer, half-fill with water and add two or three drops of essential oil.

Lemon, lavender and geranium work well, as does eucalyptus or tea tree for a more antiseptic whiff. You can add a drop of vodka or a few drops of vinegar to preserve, and spritz around to your heart's content.

For neutralizing smells you can't beat bicarbonate of soda. Simply leave some in a carton or jar; it works a treat if you've been decorating (on that note, by the way, it's more expensive but if you can opt for eco-paint you will never regret it – see www.nutshellpaints.com, www.auro.co.uk and www.farrow-ball.com).

If you must buy an air freshener, then make it one of the natural room sprays from Neal's Yard remedies or combine it with a 'bug-busting' action – get the excellent Bugs at Bay essential oil spray from www.homescents.co.uk.

Candles can make any space look romantic and intimate, but make sure you choose natural ones. It may surprise you to know that cheap candles are made with petrochemicals and can emit some pretty toxic stuff.

For excellent natural candles made from soy wax or beeswax:

- www.indigoessences.com
- www.aroma-candles.co.uk
- www.lajewellery.co.uk – for La Lumiere, a lovely organic soy candle with a hemp wick
- www.imperfectlynatural.com – for instructions on making your own beeswax candles.

Eco Cleaning Products

Back on cleaning, if you want to buy commercial products stick to the eco brands, they use plant-based surfactants which are much kinder to the environment and our skin. To list a few of my favourite companies, the bigger ones you'll find in the supermarkets and health stores include:

- www.ecover.com – always make sure you use their re-filling service, too
- www.biodegradable.biz
- www.methodproducts.co.uk
- www.greenbrands.co.uk – for Earth-friendly products
- www.daylesfordorganic.com

There are also some smaller companies who have developed some great ethical cleaning products that really work:

- www.livingclean.co.uk – make the excellent 'Budge', which really does blitz everything, naturally
- www.naturohome.co.uk – do the best orange degreaser to mop up after even the messiest roast dinners or barbecues
- www.kinetic4health.co.uk – for chlorine-free bleach
- www.naturalcollection.com – for stainless steel 'smell-busters'
- www.lemonburst.co.uk – for Pierre d'Argent, a really tough natural oven cleaner

Cleaning Kit

For cleaning materials, microfibre cloths are a truly wonderful invention because you don't usually need detergent: water alone lifts the dirt: www.e-cloth.com.

For oven mitts, cleaning gloves (which are brilliant for getting into tricky corners) and the most incredible telescopic microfibre mop: www.enjo.net.

Steam Cleaners

Don't underestimate how brilliant steam cleaning is. Ask if you can borrow one from a friend, or pick one up through Freecycle or eBay. You can transform curtains, carpets, furnishings, even cupboards and surfaces with a few hours' therapeutic blasting!

Carpets and Vacuum Cleaners

In an ideal world we'd ditch the carpets, have sustainable flooring and live happily ever after, but for the areas where you like your carpet, avoid conventional carpet-cleaning products. You know why! If you want to refresh a carpet, shake bicarbonate of soda over it and then hoover. Add a spritz or two of essential oil if you really want to rival that household name carpet-cleaner advertised on TV all those years ago!

When choosing a vacuum cleaner there are a few that use a bowl of water to catch the dust particles, but I've yet to find an affordable one. More common are the ones with Hepa filters, great if you have pets. For resources and lots more information, see www.healthy-house.co.uk.

DO-IT-YOURSELF CLEANING

You already know about using vinegar and newspaper for cleaning windows; many DIY cleaning ideas are similarly old school.

Vinegar

Use vinegar mixed with bicarbonate of soda for a really strong fizzing solution for drains. Vinegar will help prevent limescale in the loo; for around taps, soak a cotton wool pad in it, pop a plastic bag around the tap and leave for a couple of hours before washing off. You can mix it with lemon juice and water to clean surfaces and floors and, of course, de-scale kettles.

Lemons

These should be kept to the bitter end, because a used lemon will shine a ceramic sink beautifully. You can add salt to half a lemon with the flesh all used up and use it as a scouring mitt. A tiny bit of lemon peel in the cutlery tray of the dishwasher works a treat, too.

Bicarbonate of Soda

There are thousands of uses for this wonder product: it neutralizes odours, cleans plastics and removes stains from mugs and coffee parts (as a paste with a bit of water), polishes chrome, mixes with vinegar to clean loos and drains, and can be left overnight to clean the oven. It can even be used as shampoo and toothpaste (see haircare chapter). Check out Margaret Briggs' fab book *Bicarbonate of Soda*.

Essential Oils

These live up to their name in household cleaning. Tea tree is a strong anti-bacterial. Lavender is all purpose and will double up as a great massage oil, and is brilliant to dab on neat if you burn yourself on the cooker.

LAUNDRY

This is a no-brainer: you can save yourself a small fortune not buying conventional laundry products. You'll also find that your clothes last longer, no more itchy rashes and you'll be reducing your carbon footprint. Easy-peasy.

First off, let me urge you in true 'slovenly and proud of it' style to consider doing less washing. Sometimes I wear a cardigan or T-shirt for a few hours and then for whatever reason decide to get changed. My little girl has been watching too closely: she appeared in three different outfits yesterday! So, if said item is chucked over a chair or on the floor, then my zealous au pair will probably assume it's dirty and needs washing. Not so. It took me a while to cotton on to why my energy bills were so high and I always seemed to have mountains of dry washing to sort out. I have since learned to hang up my clothes or give them a bit of an airing instead. If that makes you reel back in horror, sorry, but we in the UK alone are doing 17 million washes a day. That's a scary waste of clean water, before you even start on the energy used and the damage to the environment (and our skin) from the harsh chemicals. I'm not suggesting that we all walk around in whiffy, stained clothing, but if you've worn your jeans once or twice to the pub they can handle a few more outings before they're due a wash.

Eco Detergents

If you want to switch from your conventional powder or liquid to an eco one you have lots of choices:

— www.ecover.com
— www.natural-house.co.uk

Much cheaper and more fun is to ditch the detergents altogether and opt for laundry balls or soapnuts. Both are very cheap, eco-friendly and sustainable, and there's no need for fabric softener. With laundry balls you simply pop two in the drum with the clothing. They contain ionized pellets which change the molecular structure of the water and draw off the dirt. Be sure not to overfill the machine, as the pummelling action helps the process. You can buy laundry balls from www.ecoball.com. A pack of two, complete with natural stain remover, cost around £35 but are guaranteed to do a minimum 1,000 washes.

Even cheaper and more sustainable are soapnuts. Used in India and Nepal as natural detergent for hundreds of years, they look a bit like dried-up conkers. You simply pop five or six little shells into a drawstring bag (a thin sock works even better so that none escape!) and put it in the drum. When they come into contact with water they create saponin, which is soap. You can use them three times before putting the soapnuts on the compost and refilling the little bag. You can buy a huge sack for around £5 or £6 from www.ethicstrading.com or www.inasoapnutshell.com. You can also make your soapnut liquid by simmering two cupfuls of soapnuts in hot water for around 2 minutes, straining off the liquid, frothing it up using a hand blender and adding a couple of drops of essential oil (that bit's important, they don't smell great otherwise!). This will make the most effective detergent for anything: washing the car, household surfaces – it's also a great shampoo!

Fabric Softener and Fragrance

The regular stuff is pretty hideous, but the good news is you don't need it! Eco detergents (and obviously soapnuts and laundry balls) contain no optical brighteners, phosphates or harsh detergents to create the need for softening. If you do like a fragrance, then put a couple of drops of essential oil in the fabric softener compartment, or treat yourself to the gorgeous ironing water from www.homescents.co.uk – don't worry if you're like me and you only ever opt for clothes that don't need ironing (and get the guys to do their own), the spray doesn't know! It simply works as a great natural fragrance for newly washed clothes. To soften towels, add a tablespoonful of vinegar to the softener compartment.

A Word about Whites

Both laundry balls and soapnuts will do a great job of washing the clothes, but they won't remove stubborn stains. Always treat stains first with bicarbonate of soda, or try Ecover's excellent stain remover. And if you want your whites very white, then wash them separately and add in some eco laundry bleach.

Drying

Ah, the answer here is so simple but so difficult to achieve: in an ideal world we'd all hang our washing out to dry. A great tip for white cotton, especially babies' cloth nappies, is to spritz them with lemon juice before hanging them out in the sunshine – the perfect natural bleach for even the hardiest stains!

If you don't have the luxury of a washing line but have got a rotary dryer, you can now get a special cover to save the hassle of running in and out when it rains: www.rotaire.com.

Tumble and Fall

I'm not a fan of tumble dryers, all that reverse action is not good for fabrics and they eat a hideous amount of energy.

My top tip here is to ask your granny if she still has her old-style top-loading spin dryer. I found one in a junk shop for ten quid and it has saved me a fortune in time and energy. Even after a 1400 spin in an efficient washing machine/dryer the 2-minute whizz in the spin dryer seems to manage to squeeze out a torrent of water, leaving your clothes not far off dry, then they can dry off and air for a few hours on a pulley or clothes horse.

HOUSE PLANTS

An interesting switch, I hear you say; we've been talking about ditching chemicals and looking at cleaning, laundry and how pollutants affect our health and well-being, why now are we on to aesthetics? Well, the right houseplants can be your saving grace in the pollution department. NASA scientists tell us that one peace lily can remove pollutants including formaldehyde from the air to a radius of 30 feet. Spider plants are also good, and very hardy even if you never get round to talking to them. It is advised that we have one plant for every bit of electronic equipment, which means the average girlfriend's study could start to look like Kew Gardens, but even one or two are a good start. Don't get depressed if they start to wilt, either, just replace them and be glad it's them rather than you soaking up the negative stuff!

EMFS

It's way too big a subject to get into here, and slightly off topic for the main thrust of this book, but as you're aware the holistic approach is important to me. To that end I'm just going to urge you to reduce your usage of mobile phones (and

use a protective quartz crystal device like Phoneshield: www.
phoneshield.co.uk and look at the protective products from
www.bioenergyproducts.co.uk and www.bioprotectivesystems.
co.uk). Switch off your wi-fi at night so that you can at least
get restorative sleep, and *never* have a computer or TV in your
bedroom – that room is for sleep and sex alone. Of course for
most of us we have overstuffed wardrobes in there, too, but unless you have only the one room to your flat, keep the electronic
equipment out. Especially don't sleep with anything near your
head that has a transformer – as many halogen lamps do.

Don't use your mobile phone as an alarm clock. Buy an
old style wind-up or battery one for a few quid. Most of
us are aware of the possible detrimental effects of constant
mobile phone use but we forget that cordless phones are also
a concern, in fact they can be considered worse as they are
'on duty' all the time seeking out their little receiver friends.
Certainly do not keep the mother station of a cordless phone
on your bedside table, and look into the possibility of ditching them completely and going old-style with hard wiring.
If that's not an option for you, at least look into the newer
DECT-style phones, which are said to cause less harm.

More reading on this subject:

- *Something in the Air* by Roger Coghill
- *Electromagnetic Fields – what you need to know to protect
  your health* by Laurie Tarkan
- Various articles by John Kelsey
  www.imperfectlynatural.com

LIGHT BOXES
See the chapter on Staying Well for more on seasonal affective disorder (SAD), but in short it's a really worthwhile

investment to get a light box or even some daylight simulation bulbs. Of course getting out for a walk in the fresh air is preferable, but when daylight is scarce, 20 minutes' pottering around near to a light box has an incredible effect on your well-being. See www.apollo-health.co.uk and www.litebook.com for their excellent portable light boxes, and www.wholisticresearch.com for a great range of boxes and bulbs.

Himalayan salt lamps are also a very attractive and therapeutic addition to your home. They give off a lovely orange glow and are said to ionize the air and improve sleep quality. You can also get Himalayan salt tea light holders.

- www.amazinghealth.co.uk
- www.thesaltseller.co.uk

For further resources see:

- *Imperfectly Natural Home* by Janey Lee Grace
- *Creating Sacred Space with Feng Shui* by Karen Kingston
- *Cleaning Yourself to Death* by Pat Thomas

Janey's Guide to Feng Shui and Clutter-clearing

As you're well aware, feng shui is an ancient Chinese art still used worldwide to determine auspicious sites. Sadly, for most of us the option of getting a feng shui master to determine the perfect spot for us to build a house is not a realistic option, but we can certainly apply a few of the principles in our homes.

Probably the most important thing to consider is whether the energy of your prospective (or current) home feels right. You know what it's like – some homes, big or small, expensively furnished or very simple, feel extremely welcoming and homely; others, however outwardly 'comfortable', expensively furnished or even ostentatious, feel a bit cold and creepy.

It's a great idea to find out a little about the history of the previous inhabitants of your home. We used to live in a house that had rarely been owned but had hosted mostly short-term tenants for most of its 200-year life. Consequently the walls held the experiences of hundreds of previous lives, a real mixed bag of energies! Your library or local studies centre will have directories that list, by street, the occupants of your home, sometimes going back hundreds of years.

I called in an expert who did a special ceremony to 'space clear' the whole house, and I highly recommend this if you can afford it. You can also do your own mini-'initiation' ceremony in a new home or even to refresh the energies in your existing one if it feels rather 'stuck'. Simply light a stick of white sage and 'waft it round', especially in the corners. I know it doesn't sound very technical, but believe me it really helps. It's a good idea, too, to light a candle and voice out loud your intention for your new home or for a new phase in your life.

Of course the biggest factor in how your home affects you will be how much clutter you've got. I'm not suggesting everyone must be minimalist, but some people have years' and years' worth of accumulated stuff which is blocking new energies from coming in – both metaphorically and literally. Here's one area I've really had to address in my own life. I'm a hoarder, no doubt about it, and while I absolutely know all the truths about feeling lighter and allowing opportunities to come in if you free up the space, I do find it hard to part with gifts, clothes and ornaments that have sentimental value, and pictures my children painted when they were toddlers.

My recent house move was a downsize from an over-stuffed seven-bedroom house with outbuildings into something much smaller. I can't pretend I didn't find it a harrowing experience, and in the end I simply asked a friend to come and help out.

Several weeks on and most of the boxes unpacked, and lots more thrown away, I have to say I do feel different. My best advice, if you find this hard, is think how great you'll look and feel at the end of it – and get a girlfriend to help you. We were lucky enough to have friends, who are incredibly busy with their own lives, just show up in their overalls offering help the day before we moved. It was appreciated beyond measure.

It seems only fitting that I defer here to Davina Mackail, shamanic life coach, hypnotherapist and feng shui and space-clearing expert.

Want to Look Younger? – Clear Your Clutter

'If you live surrounded by physical clutter you'll feel stuck, weighed down and old before your time.

'The nourishing energy that enters your front door will struggle to move smoothly around the rooms if it keeps encountering piles of junk stored in the hall, hidden behind doors, sofas or crowding surfaces in kids' bedrooms, the kitchen or bathroom. This slow, sluggish energy has a negative effect on you and your family. It can lead to feeling confused, blocked, lethargic, depressed and a general reluctance to move on in your lives.

'Clear your clutter and your life will start moving again. Clearing it lifts your mind, body and spirit, increases your energy and vitality and leaves you free to enjoy life, whilst looking younger, too! Remember, clutter is emotional. We collect clutter because, on some level, we don't want to let go of something. Look at your possessions with fresh eyes and ask yourself if each object reflects your love for yourself and your home. If not, it's time to bin it. By removing the old, you create fresh space for new opportunities to appear and by focusing your

intention on what you DO want your clarity of purpose will emerge.

'Intention is key. If you weed a garden and leave it, the weeds return stronger than before. But if you weed a garden and then plant it with gorgeous plants and flowers, the weeds have no room to return. Take exactly the same approach with your clutter. Make sure you know what you want to fill your newly created space with, be it more joy, more love or more money. This way you will stop the clutter returning.'

— www.askdavina.com

You know the 'If I haven't worn it for a year I never will' rule? I know it, too, but somehow I always come up with excuses about how certain garments may come around and be fashionable again. It's not an entirely daft concept: we all know that flares, puffball skirts, legwarmers and even huge shoulder pads have made a comeback, but have you noticed how the new styles are always a twist on the old, so it's never as simple as dragging your tattered old thing from behind the shelving in the wardrobe? The same applies to all our possessions: most of us have way too many pots and pans, too much furniture, ornaments, stationery, you name it! In my ripe old age I've finally learned to use the 'Do I really love it or need it?' rule. We all know the famous quote – 'Have nothing in your home that you do not know to be useful or believe to be beautiful' (William Morris). So ask yourself if you use each item or if it's beautiful, and let everything else go. If it's something you simply have no need for, then pass it on.

Presents are one tricky area. We've all been given gifts by well-meaning friends or relatives, and we can feel obliged to hang onto them. Release yourself from that pressure. Always give gifts with the intention that you allow the recipient to do whatever they will with that gift. It's the gesture that counts, after all. Similarly, don't feel you simply must use that hideous salt and pepper set just because Aunt Jemima bought it; pass it on, perhaps to the charity shop, where someone else may well treasure it. Enjoy being fabulously 'eco' with your present-giving and accept that it's now very fashionable to 're-gift' – yes, give a gift that you don't want to someone whom it may just suit. Obviously make sure it's in decent condition, but aside from that if the thought is there and it's a present fitting to the person, pass it on – we all just have to hope we don't eventually get our own gifts re-gifted back to us!

When it comes to clothes, we've already said dump it if you haven't worn it for over a year, and of course if you've lost weight or put weight on and your clothes, even decent ones, don't fit you any more, then let them go, too. The whole idea of de-junking your wardrobe definitely appeals to me, but so does buying less. I've never been one of those 'buy new clothes every season' type gals; I have a much more haphazard approach which is, quite frankly, charity-shop chic, but at least I'm ahead of my time in that it's very green to recycle – though even here it's hard to exercise control sometimes and I have found myself buying an item simply because it's a bargain.

I'd definitely recommend clothes-swap parties (see the Ethical Fashion chapter). If you're organizing one, get every-one to email with their dress size first so that you know there will be something to fit everyone – if you're a size missing you'll need to entice another friend along.

FENG SHUI – THE PLACEMENT OF OBJECTS

There is lots about this in my previous books, and in fact even when writing those I said I felt perhaps feng shui was 'so last year!' I absolutely believe in the arrangement and placement of certain objects, the clearing of energies and definitely in the whole clutter-clearing process, but I think the rather 1980s idea of simply buying a wind chime or a mirror to ward off evil is a little off the mark.

If you can afford to have a consultation with someone recommended, it's likely that he or she will check your home for geopathic stress and advise you on the best place to place certain things, such as which way your bed is facing. That can be a really important consideration. Many chronically ill people find wellness as soon as they change the position of their bed.

When it comes to possessions and your surroundings, especially things 'on show' such as paintings and ornaments, remember that your choice of these items says something about you, and sometimes we can unconsciously exacerbate a situation that we would rather avoid. It's thought that areas within the layout of your home correspond to aspects of your life. This can be quite literal and commonsense when you understand it. The Chinese call this layout the *bagua*, and you can apply the principles yourself by finding out where the rooms are that correspond to certain things such as your relationships – it's a great idea not to keep your rubbish bags in your relationship area, lest your love life is rubbish, too! In your 'wealth corner', make sure you have imagery and possessions that support financial security, such as a money plant (they look great, anyway). In the area that corresponds to your career or 'fame', have a picture that represents what you want, for example if you want to work in television, have a picture of a TV set there. You could even have a picture ripped from a magazine temporarily, or put your vision board there (see the chapter on Abundance). It doesn't matter too much what it is, it's the message it 'sends out' that counts.

A girlfriend of mine had a series of unsuccessful relationships and one-night stands until a feng shui expert pointed out that she had only pictures of lonely-looking single women throughout her home and particularly in her romance 'corner' where there was a huge painting of a sad old woman sitting alone under a tree. She replaced that picture with a more fortuitous painting of two love-birds, got a few other images that represented 'couples' around her home and, sure enough, was married within a year! Of course it may all sound a bit simplistic, but it doesn't hurt to look with fresh eyes at the messages you are perhaps unconsciously sending out into the universe. Check out the excellent book *Clear Your Clutter with Feng Shui* by Karen Kingston.

Conclusion

Girlfriends' Natural Secrets ... BEAUTY *truly comes from deep within – an ability to* LOVE *and embrace your whole self allows your* BEAUTY *to shine for all to see.* BEAUTY *comes naturally when inner peace is accomplished; no one can ignore a loving heart.*

Girlfriends' Aspirations ... To help as many people as possible to find their inner peace.

– Debs Wade, masseur, Reiki master

I hope that if you've come to the end of this book you're feeling excited about trying out some new ideas, saving some money and getting back in touch with who you really are. I hope you can now see that you certainly don't have to ditch your lipstick (or any other pampering aid) in the name of being natural, holistic and eco.

If, however, you're feeling at all overwhelmed or even guilty that you're not getting everything right, simply ditch that feeling and start with one small step. Treat yourself to a natural lipstick or a sparkly mineral powder eyeshadow, whizz up your own concoction of skincare and/or cleaning products, buy a natural deodorant or do your next laundry wash with soapnuts, and then, when you're feeling triumphantly richer and greener, move on to the next step. It's the small change/big difference approach that really gets results.

If I could pass on only one message from this book, what would it be? Well, that's easy. Of course I'm passionate about ditching the synthetic chemicals, and about juicing, eating raw and exercising regularly – but the most important message of all is that *you are already beautiful*. Yes, you. Your beauty comes from within. It may be that you have smothered it in processed foods and chemical creams so it needs a bit of a shake-up, but it's there all right. When you get in touch with who you are, when you take steps to realize that you are in control of your own happiness, you can 'unlearn' stress and you can use your own incredible mind to both heal yourself and manifest your desires. And then you will feel rich and gorgeous.

Looking great isn't only about good features, a slim body and perfect make-up, it's about the energy you radiate. We've all met women who are immaculately coiffured, botoxed up to the hilt, clearly rich, wearing expensive designer clothes, but their lipsticked mouth doesn't smile (often that's a result of too much surgery) and their eyes don't smile, either. We've all seen stick-thin models who some consider 'beautiful', but when we ask our husbands and partners, 'Be honest, do you fancy her?' the answer is often 'No way!'

In the course of my work interviewing celebrities, I have met countless actresses and stars (I won't drop names) – and many of these are world-renowned beauties – who look simply gorgeous on the silver screen, but when you sit opposite them in reality have zero sex appeal. One film star I interviewed was so 'distant' – she was in the room physically but it was as though her soul wasn't there – I really did wonder if she was a Stepford Wife or perhaps a replicant (have you seen *Bladerunner?*). And no, I don't mean Daryl Hannah – she radiates a really beautiful energy.

I have also met many actresses who are not considered classically beautiful who nevertheless have an energy that is irresistible. There are a couple of stars who are in their sixties and when they come into the BBC studios everyone, the guys and the girls, can see that they light up the room.

Stunningly 'beautiful' women can be just that, stunningly beautiful – but somehow not sexy or attractive. Can you think of a girlfriend who is clearly overweight and perhaps not 'standardly' beautiful, but boy is she sexy?! I have one girlfriend who is a strapping big girl; she eats like a horse and isn't about to stop for anyone, but you know what? She looks great naturally, she is incredibly sexy and her exuberance and joy are infectious.

If you are skimming through this book, and want to read just one chapter in detail, I'd urge it be the chapter on abundance. Your natural beauty will shine from within if you're happy and comfortable in your skin. Everything else will feel natural and you'll gravitate towards making the right choices in every area of your life. I would also urge you to remember the incredible value of sharing with other girlfriends. Share your joy, your sadness, your make-up, your beauty tips, your secrets, your money if necessary! Support each other and we will all reap the benefits of the 'natural holistic sisterhood'.

To that end, please come and join my thriving, happy forum at www.imperfectlynatural.com.

I wish you a healthy holistic natural future!

All these ripples of holistic healing will one day add up to a sea of health.

Directory

www.imperfectlynatural.com
www.janeysnaturalstore.com

Skincare
Organic Accreditation
www.bdih.de
www.ecocert.com
www.organicfarmers.org.uk
www.safecosmetics.org
www.soilassociation.co.uk
www.viridian-nutrition.com

Natural Alternatives
www.badgerbalm.com
www.balmbalm.co.uk
www.drbronner.com
www.faithinnature.co.uk
www.greenpeople.co.uk
www.inlight-online.co.uk
www.kinetic4health.co.uk
www.lavera.co.uk
www.spieziaorganics.com
www.weleda.co.uk

Smaller Suppliers
www.beyondskincare.co.uk

www.elenasnaturecollection.co.uk
www.essential-care.co.uk
www.herbfarmacy.co.uk
www.jowoodorganics.com
www.livenative.com
www.lucyrose.biz
www.lucyrussellorganics.com
www.naturalskincarecompany.com
www.purenuffstuff.co.uk
www.rawgaia.com
www.raw-ganic.com
www.sensitiveskincareco.com

Natural Soaps and Bathtime Products
www.divastores.com
www.eoco.org.uk
www.ethicalsuperstore.com
www.handmadenaturals.co.uk
www.potions.com
www.trevarnoskincare.com
www.weleda.co.uk

Moisturizing
www.coconoil.com
www.sensitiveskincareco.com

Deodorants
www.faithinnature.com
www.greenpeople.co.uk
www.thenaturalcollection.com
www.pitrok.co.uk
www.weleda.co.uk

Sunscreens
www.drhauschka.co.uk
www.purenuffstuff.co.uk
www.weleda.co.uk
www.yaoh.co.uk

Insect Repellents
www.badgerbalm.com
www.homescents.co.uk

Facial Oils
www.annemarieborlind.co.uk
www.forestsecretsskincare.com
www.greenpeople.co.uk
www.herbfarmacy.co.uk
www.inlight-online.co.uk
www.lucyrussellorganics.co.uk

Toner
www.potions.co.uk
www.tortuerouge.co.uk

Essential Oils
www.justaromatherapy.co.uk
www.potions.co.uk
www.speciallittlepeople.co.uk
www.tortuerouge.co.uk
www.wristangel.co.uk

Cosmetics
www.elysambre.nat-cos.com
www.greenpeople.co.uk

www.inikacosmetics.co.uk
www.lavera.co.uk
www.lilylolo.co.uk
www.puritycosmetics.co.uk

Teenage Skin
www.greenpeople.co.uk
www.naturalcollateral.com
www.sensitiveskincareco.com

Hair, Teeth and Nails
Natural Salons
www.abigailjames.com
www.spiritorganic.com

Colouring
www.herbatint.co.uk
www.logona.co.uk
www.naturesdream.co.uk

Natural Shampoos
www.essential-care.co.uk
www.soorganic.com
www.rawgaia.com

Hair Removal
www.moom-uk.com
www.soorganic.com

Toothpastes
www.absolutelypure.co.uk
www.fresh-network.com
www.mionegroup.com
www.organ-nics.com

Natural Nail Polish
www.allergybestbuys.co.uk
www.cultbeauty.co.uk
www.greenhands.co.uk

www.jennysnails.info
www.lucyrose.biz
www.spiritorganic.com

The Power of Fragrance
www.eoco.org.uk
www.justaromatherapy.co.uk
www.organic-courses.com
www.potions.co.uk

Exercise
www.thechimachine.co.uk
www.nianow.com
www.shaktimat.co.uk
www.uk.mbt.com
www.uknia.com
www.womensrunningnetwork.co.uk

Yoga
www.pranasanayoga.co.uk

Journey to Tranquillity
www.juicemaster.com

Dance
www.guiltypleasures.co.uk
www.uknia.com

Ethical Fashion
www.bambooclothing.co.uk
www.blindlemonvintage.co.uk
www.cielshop.co.uk
www.edunonline.com
www.ecotextile.com
www.ethical-fashions.com
www.fashion-conscience.com
www.freecycle.org

www.heavenlyanarchist.com
www.hempish.com
www.labourbehindthelabel.org
www.myvintage.co.uk
www.peopletree.co.uk
www.stylewillsaveus.com
www.vintagefashionguild.org

Casual Wear and Gym Kit
www.ascensiononline.com
www.eco-age.com
www.eco-eco.co.uk
www.gossypium.co.uk

Eco Designers
www.diva-stores.com

Jewellery
www.credjewellery.com
www.greenkarat.com
www.lajewellery.com
www.puredesigncompany.co.uk

Bags
www.bagsofchange.co.uk
www.basketbasket.co.uk
www.onyabags.co.uk
www.turtlebags.co.uk
www.zpm.com

Shoes
www.freerangers.co.uk
www.greenshoes.co.uk
www.hempish.com
www.lovethoseshoes.com
www.simpleshoes.com
www.vegshoes.co.uk

Socks
www.corrymoor.com

Dry Cleaning
www.greenearth.co.uk

Staying Well
www.abigailjames.com
www.ainsworths.com
www.allergybestbuys.com
www.the-alpha-matrix.com
www.amazinghealth.co.uk
www.apitherapy.biz
www.asphalia.co.uk
www.asyra.co.uk
www.bachcentre.com
www.baldwins.co.uk
www.bowentechnique.com
www.canceractive.com
www.consciousfood.co.uk
www.ecoflow.com
www.emofree.com
www.fht.org.uk
www.hambledonherbs.co.uk
www.haymax.biz
www.health4health.org.uk
www.healthy-house.co.uk
www.helios.co.uk
www.hypnosisaudio.com
www.indigoessences.com
www.inlight-online.com
www.innertalk.co.uk
www.ins-f.org
www.integralnutrition.co.uk
www.jolunn.co.uk
www.lemonburst.co.uk
www.liberate-online.co.uk
www.marilynglenville.com

www.marlaypractice.co.uk
www.minami-nutrition.co.uk
www.stillnessbuddy.com
www.uk-cs.co.uk
www.theunlearningfoundation.com
www.yestolife.org.uk

Colonics
www.taymount.com

Girly Things
www.angelssecret.co.uk
www.babeland.co.uk
www.billings-centre.ab.ca
www.centerjd.org/archives/studies/
BitterestPill(f).pdf
www.coco-de-mer.com
www.doula.org.uk
www.femmecup.com
www.herbalremedyshop.com
www.kegel-exercises.com
www.livenative.co.uk
www.mooncup.co.uk
www.moontimes.co.uk
www.natracare.com
www.pelvictoner.co.uk
www.secret-ceres.com
www.sexandrelationshipcourses.com
www.yesyesyes.org

Abundance
www.angeltherapy.com
www.britishdowsers.org
www.bluelotusliving.com
www.crystalgreen.co.uk

Good Food
www.aconbury.co.uk

www.amazinghealth.co.uk
www.bigbarn.co.uk
www.billygoatstuff.co.uk
www.boojabooja.com
www.cafedirect.co.uk
www.country-markets.co.uk
www.detoxyourworld.com
www.fishonline.org
www.freshandlivemama.com
www.fresh-network.com
www.gojiking.co.uk
www.groovyfood.co.uk
www.inlight-online.co.uk
www.juicemaster.com
www.justseaweed.com
www.kefir.net
www.lifescapemag.com
www.littleguru.co.uk
www.livingfood.co.uk
www.manukahoney.co.uk
www.mayanmagic.com
www.msc.org
www.naked-chocolate.com
www.naturalgreens.co.uk
www.nibchoc.com
www.radiancecleanse.com
www.therawchef.com
www.rawfairies.com
www.therawfoodcoach.com
www.rawforlife.co.uk
www.safrestaurant.co.uk
www.thesaltseller.co.uk
www.shazzie.com
www.steenbergs.co.uk
www.sunchlorella.co.uk
www.sweetfreedom.co.uk
www.sweetsensations.uk.com
www.tachyon-energy-products.com

www.vitacoco.com
www.wildmanwildfood.co.uk
www.xynergy.co.uk

Water
www.deesidewater.co.uk
www.evolutionlife.co.uk
www.waterwise.com
www.water-for-health.co.uk
www.wholistic-health.com
www.wholisticresearch.com

Kitchen Kit
www.changinghabits.com.au
www.pamperedchef.com
www.ukthermomix.com

Alcohol
www.thealcoholfreeshop.co.uk
www.lono.co.uk
www.organic-champagne.co.uk
www.vinceremos.co.uk
www.vintageroots.co.uk

Your Home
www.thecurtainexchange.net
www.drapersorganiccotton.co.uk
www.finecottoncompany.com
www.hempsolutions.co.uk
www.my-kea.co.uk
www.serenitysilk.co.uk

Cleaning
www.aroma-candles.co.uk
www.auro.co.uk
www.biodegradable.biz
www.daylesfordorganic.com
www.ecover.com

www.e-cloth.com
www.enjo.net
www.farrow-ball.com
www.greenbrands.co.uk
www.healthy-house.co.uk
www.homescents.co.uk
www.indigoessences.com
www.kinetic4health.co.uk
www.lajewellery.co.uk
www.lemonburst.co.uk
www.livingclean.co.uk
www.methodproducts.co.uk
www.naturalcollection.com
www.naturohome.co.uk
www.nutshellpaints.com

Laundry
www.ecoball.com
www.ecover.com
www.ethicstrading.com
www.homescents.co.uk
www.inasoapnutshell.com
www.natural-house.co.uk
www.rotaire.com

EMFs and Light Boxes
www.amazinghealth.co.uk
www.apollo-health.co.uk
www.bioenergyproducts.co.uk
www.litebook.com
www.phoneshield.co.uk
www.thesaltseller.co.uk
www.wholisticresearch.com

Recommended Reading

Lindsay Adness, *Change Your Life with NLP* (Selector)

Janet Balaskas, *The Water Birth Book* (Thorsons)

Margaret Briggs, *Bicarbonate of Soda* (Abbeydale Press)

Christina Brown, *The Yoga Bible: The Definitive Guide to Yoga Postures* (Godsfield Press)

Elaine Bruce, *Living Foods for Radiant Health* (Thorsons)

Deepak Chopra, *The Seven Spiritual Laws of Success* (Bantam Press)

Susan Clark, *What Really Works in Natural Health* (Bantam Press)

Brian R. Clement, *Supplements Exposed* (New Page Books)

Roger Coghill, *Something in the Air* (Coghill Research Laboratories)

Ram Dass, *Grist for the Mill* (Unity Press)

Harvey and Marilyn Diamond, *Fit for Life* (Bantam Books)

Gill Edwards, *Stepping into the Magic* (Piatkus Books)

Josephine Fairley, *The Ultimate Natural Beauty Book* (Kyle Cathie)

Ben Fletcher and Karen Pine, *The No Diet Diet: Do Something Different* (Orion)

Charlotte Gerson and Morton Walker, *The Gerson Therapy: The Amazing Juicing Programme for Cancer and Other Illnesses* (Thorsons)

Yehudi Gordon, *Birth and Beyond* (Vermilion)

Janey Lee Grace, *Imperfectly Natural Home* (Orion)

------, *Imperfectly Natural Woman* (Crown House Publishing)

Tom Graves, *Elements of Pendulum Dowsing* (Element Books)

Edward Group, *Complete Colon Cleanse* (Ulysses Press)

David R. Hamilton, PhD, *Why Kindness Is Good for You* (Hay House, 2010)

Katherine Hamnett and Matilda Lee, *Eco Chic: The Savvy Shoppers Guide to Ethical Fashion* (Gaia Books)

Louise Hay, *You Can Heal Your Life* (Hay House)

Richard Hobday, *Healing Sun* (Findhorn Press Ltd)

Tom Hodgkinson, *How to Be Free* (Penguin)

------, *How to Be Idle* (Penguin)

Carl Honore, *In Praise of Slow* (Orion)

Galina Imrie, *Always Look After Number Two* (Fotherby Press)

Oliver James, *Affluenza* (Vermilion)

Susan Jeffers, *Feel the Fear and Do It Anyway* (Vermilion)

Dr Bernard Jensen, *Dr Jensen's Guide to Better Bowel Care* (J P Tarcher/ Penguin Putnam)

Leslie Kenton, *The Raw Energy Bible* (Vermilion)

Star Khechara, *The Holistic Beauty Book* (Green Books)

Karen Kingston, *Clear Your Clutter with Feng Shui* (Piatkus Books)

------, *Creating Sacred Space with Feng Shui* (Piatkus Books)

Jay Kordich, *The Juiceman's Power of Juicing* (Morrow/Avon)

Davina MacKail, *The Dream Whisperer* (Hay House)

Steve Meyerowitz, *Sprouts, the Miracle Food: The Complete Guide to Sprouting* (Book Publishing Company)

Barbel Mohr, *Cosmic Ordering for Beginners* (Hay House)

Dr Gowri Motha and Karen Swan Macleod, *The Gentle Birth Method* (Thorsons)

Graeme Robert Munro-Hall and Lillian Munro-Hall, *Toxic Dentistry Exposed* (Browsebooks)

Anthony Robbins, *Awaken the Giant Within* (Pocket Books)

Cheryl Richardson, *The Art of Extreme Self-Care* (Hay House, 2009)

Doris Sarjeant and Karen Evans, *Hard to Swallow: The Truth about Food Additives* (Alive Books)

Shazzie, *Shazzie's Detox Delights* (Rawcreation Ltd)

------, *Detox Your World* (Rawcreation Ltd)

Laurie Tarkan, *Electromagnetic Fields – What you need to know to protect your health* (Bantam)

Pat Thomas, *Cleaning Yourself to Death* (Newleaf)

Jason Vale, *Kick the Drink ... Easily!* (Crown House Publishing)

------, *7lbs in 7 Days Super Juice Diet* (Harper Thorsons)

Michael Van Straten, *Superfoods, Superjuices, Superhealth* (Mitchell Beazley)

Doreen Virtue, *Angel Medicine* (Hay House)

------, *Angel Therapy* (Hay House)

------, *Connecting with Your Angels* (Hay House)

Dr Norman Walker, *Fresh Vegetable and Fruit Juices* (Norwalk Press)

------, *Water Can Undermine Your Health* (Norwalk Press)

Mark Williams, John Teasdale, Zindel Segal, and Jon Kabat-Zinn, *The Mindful Way Through Depression: Freeing Yourself from Chronic Unhappiness* (includes Guided Meditation Practices CD; Guilford Press)

David Wolfe, *Superfoods* (Blue Snake Books)

David Wolfe and Shazzie, *Naked Chocolate* (North Atlantic Books)

Chris Woollams, *The Rainbow Diet and How It Can Help You Beat Cancer* (Health Issues Ltd)

Valerie Ann Worwood, *The Fragrant Pharmacy* (Bantam Books)

Tonya Zavasta, *Beautiful on Raw* (BR Publishing)

CDs and DVDs

Cori Brackett, *Sweet Misery: A Poisoned World* – documentary film: you'll never go near artificial sweeteners again!

James Colquhoun, *Food Matters*

Nick Francis and Mark Francis, *Black Gold*

Janey Lee Grace and Glenn Harrold, *Creative Conception* (Hypnosis audio CD)

Marlee Matlin, *What the Bleep Do We Know?*

Jeff Nelson, *Processed People*

Ken Ryan, *Journey to Tranquillity* – a great yoga DVD

'In my profession I want to look good and age gracefully, but I want to do it without hurting animals or poisoning myself with chemicals. Thanks to Janey Lee Grace I can do both and not go broke too!!!'

- Jenny Seagrove, actress

'Janey Lee Grace has put herself on the front line of sensible and pragmatic planet-saving advice. Anyone who wants to do their bit should start here.'

- Matthew Wright, FIVE's The Wright Stuff

JOIN THE HAY HOUSE FAMILY

As the leading self-help, mind, body and spirit publisher in the UK, we'd like to welcome you to our family so that you can enjoy all the benefits our website has to offer.

 EXTRACTS from a selection of your favourite author titles

 COMPETITIONS, PRIZES & SPECIAL OFFERS Win extracts, money off, downloads and so much more

 LISTEN to a range of radio interviews and our latest audio publications

 CELEBRATE YOUR BIRTHDAY An inspiring gift will be sent your way

 LATEST NEWS Keep up with the latest news from and about our authors

 ATTEND OUR AUTHOR EVENTS Be the first to hear about our author events

 iPHONE APPS Download your favourite app for your iPhone

 HAY HOUSE INFORMATION Ask us anything, all enquiries answered

join us online at **www.hayhouse.co.uk**

 292B Kensal Road, London W10 5BE
T: 020 8962 1230 E: info@hayhouse.co.uk

We hope you enjoyed this Hay House book.
If you would like to receive a free catalogue featuring additional
Hay House books and products, or if you would like information
about the Hay Foundation, please contact:

Hay House UK Ltd
292B Kensal Road • London W10 5BE
Tel: (44) 20 8962 1230; Fax: (44) 20 8962 1239
www.hayhouse.co.uk

***

Published and distributed in the United States of America by:
Hay House, Inc. • PO Box 5100 • Carlsbad, CA 92018-5100
Tel: (1) 760 431 7695 or (1) 800 654 5126;
Fax: (1) 760 431 6948 or (1) 800 650 5115
www.hayhouse.com

***

Published and distributed in Australia by:
Hay House Australia Ltd • 18/36 Ralph Street • Alexandria, NSW 2015
Tel: (61) 2 9669 4299, Fax: (61) 2 9669 4144
www.hayhouse.com.au

***

Published and distributed in the Republic of South Africa by:
Hay House SA (Pty) Ltd • PO Box 990 • Witkoppen 2068
Tel/Fax: (27) 11 467 8904
www.hayhouse.co.za

***

Published and distributed in India by:
Hay House Publishers India • Muskaan Complex • Plot No.3
B-2• Vasant Kunj • New Delhi - 110 070
Tel: (91) 11 41761620; Fax: (91) 11 41761630
www.hayhouse.co.in

***

Distributed in Canada by:
Raincoast • 9050 Shaughnessy St • Vancouver, BC V6P 6E5
Tel: (1) 604 323 7100
Fax: (1) 604 323 2600

***

Sign up via the Hay House UK website to receive the Hay House
online newsletter and stay informed about what's going on with your
favourite authors. You'll receive bimonthly announcements
about discounts and offers, special events, product highlights,
free excerpts, giveaways, and more!
www.hayhouse.co.uk